Nursing
Calculations

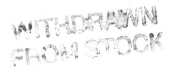

For Churchill Livingstone

Commissioning editor: Ellen Green/Alex Mathieson
Project manager: Valerie Burgess
Project editor: Valerie Dearing
Project controller: Derek Robertson
Design: Judith Wright
Promotion manager: Hilary Brown

Nursing Calculations

J. D. Gatford
Mathematics Teacher, Melbourne, Australia

R. E. Anderson
RN Intensive Care Cert DipNEd FRCNA

FIFTH EDITION

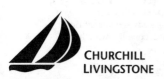

EDINBURGH LONDON NEW YORK PHILADELPHIA SYDNEY TORONTO 1998

CHURCHILL LIVINGSTONE
An imprint of Harcourt Brace and Company Limited

Churchill Livingstone, Robert Stevenson House, 1–3 Baxter's Place,
Leith Walk, Edinburgh EH1 3AF, UK

First published 1982
Second edition 1987
Third edition 1990
Fourth edition 1994
Fifth edition 1998

ISBN 0443 05966 7

British Library of Cataloguing in Publication Data
A catalogue record for this book is available from the British Library.

Library of Congress Cataloging in Publication Data
A catalog record for this book is available from the Library of Congress.

Medical knowledge is constantly changing. As new information becomes
available, changes in treatment, procedures, equipment and the use of
drugs become necessary. The authors and publishers have, as far as it is
possible, taken care to ensure that the information given in this text is
accurate and up to date. However, readers are strongly advised to confirm
that information, especially with regard to drug usage, complies with the
latest legislation and standards of practice.

Produced by Addison Wesley Longman China Limited, Hong Kong
NPCC/01

Contents

Preface to the Fifth Edition   vii

Preface to the First Edition   viii

Acknowledgements   ix

1. A review of basic calculations   1

2. Drug dosages for injection   51

3. Dosages of tablets and mixtures   63

4. Dilution and strengths of solutions   71

5. Intravenous infusion   83

6. Paediatric dosages (body weight)   97

7. Paediatric dosages (surface area)   107

8. Summary exercises   113

9. Answers   121

Preface to the Fifth Edition

The authors wish to thank those nurse educators and nurses who offered constructive criticism of the first four editions.

In this fifth edition, two new exercises have been added to the chapter 'Drug Dosages for Injection'. One of these exercises shows how estimation can be used to check whether calculated answers are within the correct range. The other exercise involves the reading of volumes of solutions drawn up in syringes.

A new exercise has also been added to the chapter 'Intravenous Infusion', where energy intakes for various infusions are to be calculated.

Drug usage has been revised and updated. Typical doses for patients are used in all calculations involving drugs. However, it must be stressed that the aim of *Nursing Calculations* is to teach relevant *arithmetical* skills: the book is *not* meant to be used as a pharmacology reference.

Further suggestions and comments are always greatly appreciated.

Melbourne 1998   J.D.G., R.E.A.

Preface to the First Edition

This book was written at the request of nurse educators and with considerable help from them. It deals with elements of the arithmetic or nursing, especially the arithmetic of basic pharmacology.

The book begins with a diagnostic test which is carefully related to a set of review exercises in basic arithmetic. Answers to the test are supplied at the back of the book, and are keyed to the corresponding review exercises.

Students should work through those exercises which correspond to errors in the diagnostic test. The other exercises may also, of course, be worked through to improve speed and accuracy.

Throughout the other chapters of the book there are adequate, well graded exercises and problems. Each chapter includes several worked examples. Answers are given to all questions.

Suggestions and comments from nurse educators and students on the scope and content of this book would be welcomed. The hope is that its relevance to nursing needs will be maintained in subsequent editions.

Melbourne 1982

J.D.G.

Acknowledgements

The authors would like to thank those nurse educators, nurses and pharmacologists from Australia, the United Kingdom and Hong Kong who provided advice and constructive criticism during the preparation of this edition.

The authors wish also to thank Mary Emmerson Law, who recommended a fifth edition; Ellen Green, for her encouragement and comments on new material; Valerie Dearing and Derek Robertson, for editing the manuscripts and page proofs; Sophie Kaliniecki, our helpful contact person in Melbourne; Aaron Richardson, for the checking of answers; and Gavin Hawkins, for computer graphics.

John Gatford wishes to thank his wife, Elaine, for related secretarial work and for continuing patience and understanding.

1. A review of basic calculations

In this chapter, a list of mathematical terms is followed by a diagnostic test. This test is designed to pinpoint those areas of your arithmetic which need revising before you commence nursing calculations.

Attempt all questions.

Answers are supplied at the back of the book, and direct you to particular exercises, according to the *errors* in your test answers.

For example, if you make an error in answering either question 1 or question 2, then you will be asked to do *Exercise 1A*. Or, if your answer to question 3 or 4 is wrong, you should do *Exercise 1B*.

Remember that this test is designed to *help* you.

Short list of mathematical terms 3

Diagnostic test 6

Multiplication by 10, 100 and 1000 10

Division by 10, 100 and 1000 12

Converting metric units 14

Comparing metric measurements 16

Multiplication of decimals 18

Diluting solutions 20

Factors 22

Simplifying fractions I 24

Simplifying fractions II 26

Rounding-off decimal numbers 28

Vulgar fraction to a decimal I 30

Vulgar fraction to a decimal II 32

Vulgar fraction to a percentage 34

Dilution ratios 36

Ratio to a percentage 38

Decimal fraction to vulgar fraction 40

Percentage to vulgar fraction 42

Mixed numbers and improper fractions 44

Multiplication of vulgar fractions 46

Division by a vulgar fraction 48

SHORT LIST OF MATHEMATICAL TERMS

Whole numbers

Whole number:
A number without fractions.
e.g. 5, 17, 438, 10 592.

Whole numbers are also known as *integers*.

Vulgar fractions

Vulgar fraction:
Also known as a common fraction.
e.g. $\frac{3}{8}$ $\frac{17}{5}$ $\frac{1}{6}$ $\frac{9}{4000}$

Numerator:
The top number in a vulgar fraction.
e.g. In the fraction $\frac{3}{8}$ the numerator is 3.

Denominator:
The bottom number in a vulgar fraction.
e.g. In the fraction $\frac{3}{8}$ the denominator is 8.

Proper and improper fractions

A *proper* fraction is a vulgar fraction in which the numerator is *smaller* than the denominator.
e.g. $\frac{1}{4}$ $\frac{5}{8}$ $\frac{11}{100}$

An *improper* fraction is a vulgar fraction in which the numerator is *larger* than the denominator.
e.g. $\frac{5}{3}$ $\frac{32}{7}$ $\frac{100}{9}$

An improper fraction can be converted to a mixed number.
e.g. $\frac{5}{3} = 1\frac{2}{3}$ $\quad \frac{32}{7} = 4\frac{4}{7}$ $\quad \frac{100}{9} = 11\frac{1}{9}$

Mixed number:
Partly a whole number, partly a fraction.

e.g. $1\frac{5}{3}$ $4\frac{1}{2}$ $10\frac{4}{5}$

A mixed number can be converted to an improper fraction.

e.g. $1\frac{5}{8} = \frac{13}{8}$ $4\frac{1}{2} = \frac{9}{2}$ $10\frac{4}{5} = \frac{54}{5}$

Decimals

Decimal:
Generally used to mean a number which includes a decimal point.
e.g. 6.35, 0.748, 0.002, 236.5

Decimal places:
Numbers to the right of the decimal point.
e.g. 6.35 has 2 decimal places
     0.748 has 3 decimal places
     0.002 has 3 decimal places
     236.5 has 1 decimal place.

Place value (in decimals):
To the right of the decimal point are tenths, hundredths, thousandths, etc...
e.g. In the number 0.962, there are 9 tenths, 6 hundredths and 2 thousandths.

Percentages

Percentage:
Number of parts per hundred parts.
e.g. 14% means 14 parts per 100 parts
     2.5% means 2.5 parts per 100 parts.
A percentage may be less than 1%.
e.g. 0.3% = 0.3 parts per 100 = 3 parts per 1000
     0.04% = 0.04 parts per 100 = 4 parts per 10 000.

Other terms

Divisor:
The number by which you are dividing.
e.g. In the division $495 \div 15$, the divisor is 15.

Factors:
When a number is divided by one of its **factors**, the answer is a whole number (i.e. there is no remainder).
e.g.   The factors of 12 are 1, 2, 3, 4, 6 and 12.
       The factors of 20 are 1, 2, 4, 5, 10 and 20.
       The number 1 is a factor of *every* number.

Common factors:
Two different numbers may have **common factors**; factors which are *common* to both numbers.
e.g. 1, 2 and 4 are the common factors of 12 and 20.

Evaluate:
Calculate; find the value. The answer will be a number.

Simplify:
Write as simply as possible.

Commonly used SI (metric) prefixes

Prefix	Symbol	Factor	Example
mega	M	1 000 000	2.5 megaunits (Mu) = 2 500 000 units
kilo	k	1000	3 kilograms (kg) = 3000 grams
milli	m	0.001 (thousandth)	5 millilitres (mL) = 0.005 L = $\frac{5}{1000}$ litre
micro	μ^*	0.000 001 (millionth)	40 micrograms = 0.000 040 g = $\frac{40}{1\,000\,000}$ gram

*Always write 'micro' in full. Using 'μ' can cause errors.**

DIAGNOSTIC TEST

1 *Multiply*
  a 83 × 10   **b** 83 × 100   **c** 83 × 1000

2 *Multiply*
  a 0.0258 × 10   **b** 0.0258 × 100
  c 0.0258 × 1000

3 *Divide. Write answers as decimals.*
  a 3.78 ÷ 10   **b** 3.78 ÷ 100   **c** 3.78 ÷ 1000

4 *Divide. Write answers as decimals.*
  a $\frac{569}{10}$ **b** $\frac{569}{100}$ **c** $\frac{569}{1000}$

5 *Complete*
  a 1 gram   = ... milligrams
  b 1 milligram = ... micrograms
  c 1 litre   = ... millitres

Write answers to 6, 7 and 8 in decimal form:

6 a *Change 0.78 grams to milligrams*

  b *Change 34 milligrams to grams*

7 a *Change 0.086 mg to micrograms*

  b *Change 294 micrograms to mg*

8 a *Change 2.4 litres to millilitres*

  b *Change 965 millilitres to litres*

9 a *Change 0.07 L to mL*

  b *Change 0.007 L to mL*

  c *Which is larger: 0.07 L or 0.007 L?*

Check your answers on p 118

10 a *Convert 0.045 g to mg*

   b *Convert 0.45 g to mg*

   c *Which is heavier: 0.045 g or 0.45 g?*

11 *Evaluate (multiply)*
   a 9×3 **b** 0.9×3
   c 0.9×0.3 **d** 0.09×0.03

12 *Evaluate (multiply)*
   a 78×6 **b** 7.8×0.6
   c 0.78×6 **d** 7.8×0.06

13 *Calculate the volume of distilled water which must be added to 175 mL of stock solution to make 850 mL of diluted solution.*

14 *Calculate the volume of distilled water which must be added to 350 mL of stock solution to make $2\frac{1}{2}$ litres of diluted solution.*

15 *Which of the numbers 2, 3, 5, 6, 7, 9, 11 are **factors** of 126?*

16 *Simplify ('cancel down')*
   a $\frac{16}{24}$ **b** $\frac{56}{72}$

17 *Simplify*
   a $\frac{45}{600}$ **b** $\frac{175}{400}$

18 *Simplify*
   a $\frac{40}{50}$ **b** $\frac{60}{90}$ **c** $\frac{90}{150}$

19 *Simplify*
   a $\frac{350}{500}$ **b** $\frac{1200}{1500}$ **c** $\frac{1600}{4000}$

20 *Round-off each number correct to **one** decimal place*
   a 0.68   **b** 1.82   **c** 0.35

Check your answers on p 118

21 *Write each number correct to **two** decimal places*
   a 0.374   **b** 2.625   **c** 0.516

22 *Write each number correct to **three** decimal places*
   a 1.6081   **b** 0.5698   **c** 2.6565

23 *Change to exact decimal equivalents*
   a $\dfrac{5}{8}$ **b** $\dfrac{9}{20}$ **c** $\dfrac{17}{25}$ **d** $\dfrac{31}{40}$

24 *Change to decimals correct to **one** decimal place*
   a $\dfrac{1}{6}$ **b** $\dfrac{3}{7}$ **c** $\dfrac{7}{9}$

25 *Change to decimals correct to **two** decimal places*
   a $\dfrac{5}{7}$ **b** $\dfrac{5}{9}$

26 *Change to decimals correct to **three** decimal places*
   a $\dfrac{7}{30}$ **b** $\dfrac{59}{70}$

27 *Change to a percentage*
   a $\dfrac{3}{4}$ **b** $\dfrac{13}{20}$ **c** $\dfrac{8}{25}$

28 *Change to a percentage*
   a $\dfrac{1}{3}$ **b** $\dfrac{5}{8}$ **c** $\dfrac{5}{9}$

29 *Change these ratios to the form 1 in x*
   a 1:4   **b** 1:20

30 *Change these ratios to the form 1:y*
   a 1 in 4   **b** 1 in 30

31 *How much stock solution is present in 600 mL of solution if the dilution ratio is 1 in 3?*

32 *How much stock solution is present in 400 mL of solution if the dilution ratio is 1:4?*

Check your answers on p 118–9

33 *Change each ratio to a percentage*
   a 1 in 5   **b** 1 in 50
   c 1 in 500   **d** 1 in 5000

34 *Change to a vulgar fraction and simplify where possible*
   a 0.3   **b** 0.6   **c** 0.8

35 *Change to a vulgar fraction and simplify where possible*
   a 0.55   **b** 0.72   **c** 0.68   **d** 0.09

36 *Change to a vulgar fraction and simplify where possible*
   a 6%   **b** 43%   **c** 75%

37 *Change to a vulgar fraction and simplify if possible*
   a 0.7%   **b** 0.03%   **c** 0.05%

38 *Change to a vulgar fraction and simplify if possible*
   a $\frac{1}{2}$ %   **b** $5\frac{1}{2}$ %   **c** $17\frac{1}{2}$ %

39 *Change to mixed numbers*
   a $\frac{17}{2}$ **b** $\frac{67}{3}$ **c** $\frac{113}{5}$

40 *Change to improper fractions*
   a $2\frac{3}{4}$ **b** $12\frac{5}{6}$ **c** $28\frac{2}{5}$

41 *Multiply. Simplify where possible*
   a $\frac{2}{3} \times \frac{5}{6}$ **b** $\frac{5}{8} \times \frac{12}{7}$ **c** $\frac{9}{10} \times \frac{4}{9}$

42 *Divide. Simplify where possible*
   a $\frac{1}{3} \div \frac{1}{5}$ **b** $\frac{3}{7} \div \frac{3}{5}$ **c** $\frac{5}{8} \div \frac{7}{10}$

Check your answers on p 119

MULTIPLICATION BY 10, 100 AND 1000

Example

i 0.36 × 10   *ii 0.36 × 100*   *iii 0.36 × 1000*

Long method

i   0.36
   × 10
   ‾‾‾‾‾
   3.60

ii   0.36
   × 100
   ‾‾‾‾‾
   36.00

iii   0.36
   × 1000
   ‾‾‾‾‾
   360.00

Short method

  i 0.36 × 10   = 3.6 = 3.6

 ii 0.36 × 100   = 36. = 36

iii 0.36 × 1000 = 360. = 360

Notes

• use zeros to make up places, where necessary.
• if the answer is a whole number, the decimal point may be omitted.

Summary of short method

To multiply by	Move the decimal point
10	1 place right
100	2 places right
1000	3 places right

Exercise 1A *Multiply*

1 0.68×10
0.68×100
0.68×1000

2 0.975×10
0.975×100
0.975×1000

3 3.7×10
3.7×100
3.7×1000

4 5.62×10
5.62×100
5.62×1000

5 77×10
77×100
77×1000

6 825×10
825×100
825×1000

7 0.2×10
0.2×100
0.2×1000

8 0.046×10
0.046×100
0.046×1000

9 0.0147×10
0.0147×100
0.0147×1000

10 0.006×10
0.006×100
0.006×1000

11 3.76×10
3.76×100
3.76×1000

12 0.639×10
0.639×100
0.639×1000

13 0.075×10
0.075×100
0.075×1000

14 0.08×10
0.08×100
0.08×1000

15 0.003×10
0.003×100
0.003×1000

16 0.0505×10
0.0505×100
0.0505×1000

Check your answers on p 121

DIVISION BY 10, 100 AND 1000

Example A   *Short method*

i   *37.8 ÷ 10*   i $37.8 \div 10 = 3.\overset{\frown}{7}8$

ii *37.8 ÷ 100*   ii $37.8 \div 100 = 0.\overset{\frown}{3}78$

iii *37.8 ÷ 1000*   iii $37.8 \div 1000 = 0.\overset{\frown}{0}378$

Notes

• use zeros to make up places, where necessary.
• write a zero before the decimal point (for numbers less than one).

Example B

A division may be written as a fraction.

Evaluate   i $\dfrac{0.984}{10}$ i $\dfrac{0.984}{10} = 0.0984$

ii $\dfrac{0.984}{100}$ ii $\dfrac{0.984}{100} = 0.009\,84$

iii $\dfrac{0.984}{1000}$ iii $\dfrac{0.984}{1000} = 0.000\,984$

Summary of short method

To divide by	Move the decimal point
10	1 place left
100	2 places left
1000	3 places left

Exercise 1B   *Divide. Write answers as decimals.*

1 $98.4 \div 10$
$98.4 \div 100$
$98.4 \div 1000$

2 $5.91 \div 10$
$5.91 \div 100$
$5.91 \div 1000$

3 $2.6 \div 10$
$2.6 \div 100$
$2.6 \div 1000$

4 $307 \div 10$
$307 \div 100$
$307 \div 1000$

5 $82 \div 10$
$82 \div 100$
$82 \div 1000$

6 $7 \div 10$
$7 \div 100$
$7 \div 1000$

7 $3 \div 10$
$3 \div 100$
$3 \div 1000$

8 $7.5 \div 10$
$7.5 \div 100$
$7.5 \div 1000$

9 $\dfrac{68}{10}$

$\dfrac{68}{100}$

$\dfrac{68}{1000}$

10 $\dfrac{2.29}{10}$

$\dfrac{2.29}{100}$

$\dfrac{2.29}{1000}$

11 $\dfrac{51.4}{10}$

$\dfrac{51.4}{100}$

$\dfrac{51.4}{1000}$

12 $\dfrac{916}{10}$

$\dfrac{916}{100}$

$\dfrac{916}{1000}$

13 $\dfrac{67.2}{10}$

$\dfrac{67.2}{100}$

$\dfrac{67.2}{1000}$

14 $\dfrac{387}{10}$

$\dfrac{387}{100}$

$\dfrac{387}{1000}$

15 $\dfrac{8.94}{10}$

$\dfrac{8.94}{100}$

$\dfrac{8.94}{1000}$

16 $\dfrac{0.707}{10}$

$\dfrac{0.707}{100}$

$\dfrac{0.707}{1000}$

Check your answers on p 121

CONVERTING METRIC UNITS

Memorise

> 1 gram (g) = 1000 milligram (mg)
> 1 milligram (mg) = 1000 microgram (µg)
> 1 litre (L) = 1000 millilitre (mL)

Example A *Change 0.67 grams to mg*

$$0.67 \text{ g} = 0.67 \times 1000 \text{ mg}$$
$$= 670 \text{ mg}$$

Example B *Change 23 mg to grams*

$$23 \text{ mg} = 23 \div 1000 \text{ g}$$
$$= 0.023 \text{ g}$$

Example C *Change 0.075 mg to micrograms*

$$0.075 \text{ mg} = 0.075 \times 1000 \text{ microgram}$$
$$= 75 \text{ microgram}$$

Note
It is better to write the word micrograms than use the symbol μg.

Example D *Change 185 micrograms to mg*

$$185 \text{ micrograms} = 185 \div 1000 \text{ mg}$$
$$= 0.185 \text{ mg}$$

Example E *Change 1.3 litres to mL*

$$1.3 \text{ litres} = 1.3 \times 1000 \text{ mL}$$
$$= 1300 \text{ mL}$$

Example F *Change 850 mL to litres*

$$850 \text{ mL} = 850 \div 1000 \text{ litre}$$
$$= 0.85 \text{ litre}$$

Exercise 1C   *Write all answers in decimal form.*

Change to milligrams

1 4 g	**3** 0.69 g	**5** 0.035 g	**7** 0.655 g
2 8.7 g	**4** 0.02 g	**6** 0.006 g	**8** 4.28 g

Change to grams

9 6000 mg	**11** 865 mg	**13** 70 mg	**15** 5 mg
10 7250 mg	**12** 95 mg	**14** 2 mg	**16** 125 mg

Change to micrograms

17 0.195 mg	**20** 0.075 mg	**23** 0.625 mg
18 0.6 mg	**21** 0.08 mg	**24** 0.098 mg
19 0.75 mg	**22** 0.001 mg	

Change to milligrams

25 825 microgram	**29** 10 microgram
26 750 microgram	**30** 5 microgram
27 65 microgram	**31** 200 microgram
28 95 microgram	**32** 30 microgram

Change to millilitres

33 2 litre	**36** $4\frac{1}{2}$ litre	**39** 0.8 litre
34 30 litre	**37** 1.6 litre	**40** 0.75 litre
35 $1\frac{1}{2}$ litre	**38** 2.24 litre	

Change to litres

41 4000 mL	**43** 625 mL	**45** 95 mL	**47** 5 mL
42 10 000 mL	**44** 350 mL	**46** 60 mL	**48** 2 mL

Check your answers on p 121–2

Comparing metric measurements

Example A

i   Change 0.4 L to mL

ii   Change 0.04 L to mL

iii   Which is larger: 0.4 L or 0.04 L?

> *1 litre = 1000 mL*

i   0.4 L   = 0.4 × 1000 mL   = 400 mL

ii   0.04 L = 0.04 × 1000 mL = 40 mL

iii   0.4 L is larger than 0.04 L

Example B

i   Convert 4.3 kg to grams

ii   Convert 4.03 kg to grams

iii   Which is heavier: 4.3 kg or 4.03 kg?

> *1 kg = 1000 g*

i   4.3 kg   = 4.3 × 1000 g   = 4300 g

ii   4.03 kg = 4.03 × 1000 g = 4030 g

iii   4.3 kg is heavier than 4.03 kg

Exercise 1D   *Change each given measurement to the smaller unit required. Then (c) choose the larger of the two **given** measurements.*

Change each measurement to millilitres (mL); choose the larger volume.

				Larger
1 a 0.1 L	**b** 0.01 L			**c**
2 a 0.003 L	**b** 0.3 L			**c**
3 a 0.05 L	**b** 0.005 L			**c**
4 a 0.047 L	**b** 0.47 L			**c**

Convert each measurement to milligrams (mg); choose the larger mass (or weight).

5 a 0.4 g	**b** 0.004 g	**c**
6 a 0.06 g	**b** 0.6 g	**c**
7 a 0.07 g	**b** 0.007 g	**c**
8 a 0.63 g	**b** 0.063 g	**c**

Rewrite each measurement in micrograms (µg); choose the bigger mass (or weight).

9 a 0.002 mg	**b** 0.02 mg	**c**
10 a 0.9 mg	**b** 0.09 mg	**c**
11 a 0.001 mg	**b** 0.1 mg	**c**
12 a 0.58 mg	**b** 0.058 mg	**c**

Change each measurement to grams (g); choose the heavier mass (or weight).

13 a 1.5 kg	**b** 1.05 kg	**c**
14 a 2.08 kg	**b** 2.8 kg	**c**
15 a 0.95 kg	**b** 0.095 kg	**c**
16 a 3.35 kg	**b** 3.5 kg	**c**

Check your answers on p 122

MULTIPLICATION OF DECIMALS

Note
d.p. is used in the examples to stand for decimal places.

Example A *Evaluate*

a 8×4
b 0.8×4
c 0.8×0.4
d 0.08×0.04

a $8 \times 4 = 32$
b $0.8 \times 4 = 3.2$

    ↑ ↖ ↖
  1 d.p. + 0 d.p. ⇒ 1 d.p.

c $0.8 \times 0.4 = 0.32$

  ↗ ↑ ↖
  1 d.p. + 1 d.p. ⇒ 2 d.p.

d $0.08 \times 0.04 = 0.0032$

  ↗ ↑ ↑
  2 d.p. + 2 d.p. ⇒ 4 d.p.

Example B *Evaluate*

a 67×4
b 6.7×0.4
c 0.67×4
d 6.7×0.04

a $67 \times 4 = 268$
b $6.7 \times 0.4 = 2.68$

  ↗ ↑ ↖
  1 d.p. + 1 d.p. ⇒ 2 d.p.

c $0.67 \times 4 = 2.68$

  ↗ ↑ ↖
  2 d.p. + 0 d.p. ⇒ 2 d.p.

d $6.7 \times 0.04 = 0.268$

  ↗ ↑ ↖
  1 d.p. + 2 d.p. ⇒ 3 d.p.

Example C *Evaluate*

a 16×12
b 1.6×1.2
c 0.16×0.12
d 0.016×1.2

a $16 \times 12 = 192$
b $1.6 \times 1.2 = 1.92$
c $0.16 \times 0.12 = 0.0192$
d $0.016 \times 1.2 = 0.0192$

Exercise 1E   *Evaluate*

1 9×5

0.9×5

0.9×0.5

9×0.05

2 2×7

0.2×0.7

0.2×0.07

0.02×0.07

3 3×4

3×0.04

0.3×0.4

0.03×0.04

4 6×6

0.6×0.6

0.06×0.06

0.6×0.006

5 7×8

0.7×8

0.7×0.8

0.07×0.08

6 17×6

1.7×6

0.17×6

0.17×0.6

7 19×8

19×0.8

0.19×0.8

1.9×0.08

8 23×2

2.3×0.2

2.3×0.02

2.3×0.002

9 29×5

0.29×5

2.9×0.5

29×0.05

10 31×3

3.1×0.3

0.31×0.03

31×0.003

11 37×9

3.7×9

3.7×0.09

0.37×0.09

12 41×7

0.41×0.7

0.41×0.07

4.1×0.7

13 48×4

0.48×0.04

48×0.004

0.048×0.4

14 56×11

5.6×1.1

0.56×0.11

56×0.011

15 64×12

6.4×0.12

0.64×0.12

0.064×1.2

Check your answers on p 123

DILUTING SOLUTIONS

Stock solutions must often be diluted to obtain the strength required for a patient's treatment.

Dilution is usually done by mixing stock solution with distilled water.

Example

Calculate the volume of distilled water which must be added to 375 mL of stock solution to make 3 litres of diluted solution.

3 litres = 3000 mL

$$
\begin{array}{r}
3000 \\
375\ - \\
\hline
2625
\end{array}
$$

mL of distilled water

Exercise 1F   *Calculate the amount of distilled water which must be added to the stock solution to make up the total volume required.*

	Total volume required	Volume of stock solution		Total volume required	Volume of stock solution
1	600 mL	100 mL	16	2 litres	350 mL
2	600 mL	150 mL	17	2 litres	425 mL
3	600 mL	75 mL	18	2 litres	215 mL
4	750 mL	250 mL	19	$1\frac{1}{2}$ litres	150 mL
5	750 mL	125 mL	20	$1\frac{1}{2}$ litres	175 mL
6	750 mL	275 mL	21	$1\frac{1}{2}$ litres	235 mL
7	1000 mL	200 mL	22	$3\frac{1}{2}$ litres	800 mL
8	1000 mL	150 mL	23	$3\frac{1}{2}$ litres	650 mL
9	1000 mL	85 mL	24	$3\frac{1}{2}$ litres	195 mL
10	1200 mL	250 mL	25	3.2 litres	350 mL
11	1200 mL	165 mL	26	3.2 litres	475 mL
12	1200 mL	375 mL	27	3.2 litres	235 mL
13	1 litre	180 mL	28	4.5 litres	150 mL
14	1 litre	225 mL	29	4.5 litres	510 mL
15	1 litre	45 mL	30	4.5 litres	625 mL

Check your answers on p 123

FACTORS

Many calculations involve the simplifying (or 'cancelling down') of fractions.

This requires a knowledge of *factors*. When a number is divided by one of its factors, the answer is a whole number (i.e. there is no remainder).

Example   *Which of the numbers 2, 3, 5, 7, 11 are factors of 154?*

$$2\overline{)154} \qquad 3\overline{)154} \qquad 5\overline{)154} \qquad 7\overline{)154} \qquad 11\overline{)154}$$
$$77 \qquad\quad 51\tfrac{1}{3} \qquad\quad 30\tfrac{4}{5} \qquad\quad 22 \qquad\qquad 14$$

∴ 2, 7 and 11 are factors of 154.

Notes
- these are not the ONLY factors of 154.
- the numbers can, of course, be checked mentally!

Exercise 1G   *Which of the numbers in Column B are factors of the number (opposite) in Column A?*

	A	B
1	20	2, 3, 4, 5, 7, 8
2	36	3, 4, 5, 10, 12, 16
3	45	3, 5, 7, 11, 12, 15
4	56	2, 5, 8, 11, 14, 16
5	60	3, 4, 8, 12, 15, 20
6	72	3, 4, 6, 12, 15, 18
7	75	3, 5, 7, 11, 15, 25
8	85	3, 5, 9, 11, 15, 17
9	96	3, 8, 12, 14, 16, 24
10	100	3, 5, 8, 20, 25, 40
11	108	4, 7, 9, 12, 16, 18
12	120	3, 5, 9, 12, 15, 16
13	135	3, 5, 7, 9, 11, 15
14	144	4, 8, 12, 16, 18, 24
15	150	4, 5, 9, 12, 15, 25
16	165	3, 5, 7, 9, 11, 15
17	175	3, 5, 7, 9, 11, 15
18	180	4, 8, 12, 15, 16, 25
19	192	4, 6, 8, 12, 15, 16
20	210	4, 6, 9, 12, 14, 15

Check your answers on p 124

SIMPLIFYING FRACTIONS I

To simplify (or 'cancel down') a fraction, divide the numerator *and* the denominator by the *same* number. This number is called a *common factor.*

Example A   *Simplify $\dfrac{36}{48}$*

$$\frac{36}{48} = \frac{3}{4} \qquad \left[\begin{array}{l} \text{after dividing numerator and} \\ \text{denominator by 12} \end{array}\right]$$

Or this may be done in two or more steps:

$$\frac{36}{48} = \frac{18}{24} \qquad \left[\begin{array}{l} \text{dividing numerator and} \\ \text{denominator by 2} \end{array}\right]$$

$$= \frac{9}{12} \qquad \left[\begin{array}{l} \text{again dividing numerator and} \\ \text{denominator by 2} \end{array}\right]$$

$$= \frac{3}{4} \qquad \left[\begin{array}{l} \text{dividing numerator and} \\ \text{denominator by 3} \end{array}\right]$$

Note
$2 \times 2 \times 3 = 12.$

Example B   *Simplify $\dfrac{125}{225}$*

$$\frac{125}{225} = \frac{25}{45} \qquad \left[\begin{array}{l} \text{dividing numerator and} \\ \text{denominator by 5} \end{array}\right]$$

$$= \frac{5}{9} \qquad \left[\begin{array}{l} \text{again dividing numerator and} \\ \text{denominator by 5} \end{array}\right]$$

Exercise 1H

Part i   *Simplify ('cancel down')*

1 $\frac{8}{12}$ 6 $\frac{15}{21}$ 11 $\frac{28}{32}$ 16 $\frac{14}{42}$ 21 $\frac{36}{56}$

2 $\frac{10}{14}$ 7 $\frac{20}{24}$ 12 $\frac{22}{33}$ 17 $\frac{30}{45}$ 22 $\frac{48}{60}$

3 $\frac{6}{16}$ 8 $\frac{20}{25}$ 13 $\frac{15}{35}$ 18 $\frac{42}{48}$ 23 $\frac{52}{64}$

4 $\frac{9}{18}$ 9 $\frac{12}{28}$ 14 $\frac{32}{36}$ 19 $\frac{36}{50}$ 24 $\frac{21}{70}$

5 $\frac{15}{20}$ 10 $\frac{9}{30}$ 15 $\frac{16}{40}$ 20 $\frac{25}{55}$ 25 $\frac{32}{72}$

Part ii   *Simplify ('cancel down')*

1 $\frac{75}{150}$ 5 $\frac{125}{250}$ 9 $\frac{30}{225}$ 13 $\frac{125}{200}$ 17 $\frac{175}{225}$

2 $\frac{75}{200}$ 6 $\frac{125}{300}$ 10 $\frac{40}{175}$ 14 $\frac{375}{500}$ 18 $\frac{225}{300}$

3 $\frac{75}{250}$ 7 $\frac{125}{400}$ 11 $\frac{45}{150}$ 15 $\frac{275}{400}$ 19 $\frac{425}{600}$

4 $\frac{75}{300}$ 8 $\frac{125}{500}$ 12 $\frac{60}{375}$ 16 $\frac{100}{225}$ 20 $\frac{325}{750}$

Check your answers on p 124

SIMPLIFYING FRACTIONS II

Example A

Simplify $\dfrac{900}{1500}$

$\dfrac{900}{1500} = \dfrac{9}{15}$ $\left[\begin{array}{l}\text{dividing numerator and}\\ \text{denominator by 100}\end{array}\right]$

$\quad\quad = \dfrac{3}{5}$ $\left[\begin{array}{l}\text{dividing numerator and}\\ \text{denominator by 3}\end{array}\right]$

Example B

Simplify $\dfrac{1400}{4000}$

$\dfrac{1400}{4000} = \dfrac{14}{40}$ $\left[\begin{array}{l}\text{dividing numerator and}\\ \text{denominator by 100}\end{array}\right]$

$\quad\quad = \dfrac{7}{20}$ $\left[\begin{array}{l}\text{dividing numerator and}\\ \text{denominator by 2}\end{array}\right]$

Exercise 1I *Divide numerator **and** denominator by 10 or 100 or 1000. Then simplify further if possible.*

1 $\frac{30}{50}$ 10 $\frac{120}{160}$ 19 $\frac{400}{600}$ 28 $\frac{1400}{2500}$

2 $\frac{40}{60}$ 11 $\frac{100}{160}$ 20 $\frac{450}{600}$ 29 $\frac{2000}{2500}$

3 $\frac{60}{80}$ 12 $\frac{60}{160}$ 21 $\frac{540}{600}$ 30 $\frac{1750}{2500}$

4 $\frac{50}{120}$ 13 $\frac{200}{300}$ 22 $\frac{600}{800}$ 31 $\frac{2500}{3000}$

5 $\frac{80}{120}$ 14 $\frac{120}{300}$ 23 $\frac{750}{800}$ 32 $\frac{500}{3000}$

6 $\frac{100}{120}$ 15 $\frac{270}{300}$ 24 $\frac{320}{800}$ 33 $\frac{450}{3000}$

7 $\frac{130}{150}$ 16 $\frac{300}{500}$ 25 $\frac{1000}{1500}$ 34 $\frac{1500}{4000}$

8 $\frac{100}{150}$ 17 $\frac{450}{500}$ 26 $\frac{800}{1500}$ 35 $\frac{1200}{4000}$

9 $\frac{60}{150}$ 18 $\frac{120}{500}$ 27 $\frac{1250}{1500}$ 36 $\frac{2750}{4000}$

Check your answers on p 125

ROUNDING-OFF DECIMAL NUMBERS

Rounding-off to *one* decimal place

Method
- If the *second* decimal place is *5 or more* then *add one* to the first decimal place.
- If the second decimal place is *less than* 5 then leave the first decimal place as it is.

Example A

Write   i 0.62   ii 1.75   iii 3.49 correct to one decimal place

i 0.6 ② ≈ 0.6   ii 1.7 ⑤ ≈ 1.8   iii 3.4 ⑨ ≈ 3.5

[The symbol ≈ stands for *is approximately equal to*]

Rounding-off to *two* decimal places

Method
If the *third* decimal place is *5 or more* then *add one* to the second decimal place. If the third decimal place is *less than* 5 then leave the second decimal place as it is.

Example B

Write   i 0.827   ii 0.694   iii 2.145 correct to two decimal places

i 0.82 ⑦ ≈ 0.83   ii 0.69 ④ ≈ 0.69   iii 2.14 ⑤ ≈ 2.15

Rounding-off to *three* decimal places

Method
- If the *fourth* decimal place is *5 or more* then *add one* to the third decimal place.
- If the fourth decimal place is *less than* 5 then leave the third decimal place as it is.

Example C

Write   i 0.7854   ii 1.5968   iii 0.9705 correct to three decimal places

i 0.785 ④ ≈ 0.785   ii 1.596 ⑧ ≈ 1.597   iii 0.970 ⑤ ≈ 0.971

Exercise 1J

Part i *Write each number correct to ONE decimal place.*

1 0.93	**5** 0.58	**9** 2.37	**13** 1.06
2 0.47	**6** 0.96	**10** 1.09	**14** 2.98
3 0.85	**7** 1.57	**11** 0.16	**15** 1.02
4 0.69	**8** 1.22	**12** 2.65	**16** 0.75

Part ii *Write each number correct to TWO decimal places.*

1 0.333	**5** 0.142	**9** 2.714	**13** 0.625
2 1.667	**6** 0.125	**10** 1.285	**14** 0.777
3 0.875	**7** 0.916	**11** 0.636	**15** 2.428
4 0.833	**8** 1.571	**12** 0.222	**16** 1.857

Part iii *Write each number correct to THREE decimal places.*

1 0.4863	**5** 1.5288	**9** 0.8155	**13** 3.0909
2 0.9547	**6** 0.3113	**10** 1.1196	**14** 0.1645
3 0.6060	**7** 2.8585	**11** 0.1652	**15** 2.7801
4 1.4145	**8** 0.1699	**12** 2.9625	**16** 1.7575

Check your answers on p 125

VULGAR FRACTION TO A DECIMAL I

Some vulgar fractions have *exact* decimal equivalents; other vulgar fractions have only *approximate* decimal equivalents. The fractions in this exercise have *exact* decimal equivalents.

Example A

Change $\frac{2}{5}$ to a decimal

Method
Divide the numerator by the denominator.

$$5\overline{)2.0} \qquad \leftarrow \text{Write as many zeros as you need}$$
$$\underline{0.4}$$

$$\therefore \ \frac{2}{5} = 0.4$$

Example B

Change $\frac{3}{8}$ to a decimal

$$8\overline{)3.000} \qquad \leftarrow \text{Write as many zeros as you need}$$
$$\underline{0.375}$$

Example C

Change $\frac{3}{20}$ to a decimal

$$10\overline{)3}$$
$$2\overline{)0.30} \quad \left[\begin{array}{l} \text{divide by 10} \\ \text{and then 2} \\ \text{since } 10 \times 2 = 20 \end{array} \right] \quad or \quad \frac{3}{20} = \frac{15}{100}$$
$$\underline{0.15} \qquad\qquad\qquad\qquad\qquad\qquad = 0.15$$

Example D

Change $\frac{14}{25}$ to a decimal

$$5\overline{)14.0}$$
$$5\overline{)\ 2.80} \quad \left[\begin{array}{l} \text{divide by 5} \\ \text{and then 5 again} \\ \text{since } 5 \times 5 = 25 \end{array} \right] \quad or \quad \frac{14}{25} = \frac{56}{100}$$
$$\underline{0.56} \qquad\qquad\qquad\qquad\qquad\qquad = 0.56$$

Exercise 1K   *Change each fraction to a decimal. All of these fractions have exact decimal equivalents. Refer to examples A and B.*

1 $\frac{1}{2}$ 3 $\frac{3}{4}$ 5 $\frac{3}{5}$ 7 $\frac{1}{8}$

2 $\frac{1}{4}$ 4 $\frac{1}{5}$ 6 $\frac{4}{5}$ 8 $\frac{7}{8}$

Change each fraction to a decimal. All of these fractions have exact decimal equivalents. Refer to examples C and D.

9 $\frac{1}{20}$ 13 $\frac{1}{25}$ 17 $\frac{1}{40}$ 21 $\frac{1}{50}$

10 $\frac{7}{20}$ 14 $\frac{8}{25}$ 18 $\frac{9}{40}$ 22 $\frac{43}{50}$

11 $\frac{13}{20}$ 15 $\frac{17}{25}$ 19 $\frac{11}{40}$ 23 $\frac{1}{80}$

12 $\frac{19}{20}$ 16 $\frac{22}{25}$ 20 $\frac{27}{40}$ 24 $\frac{61}{80}$

Check your answers on p 126

VULGAR FRACTION TO A DECIMAL II

The fractions in this exercise have only *approximate* decimal equivalents.

Example A

Change $\frac{4}{7}$ to a decimal correct to ONE decimal place

$$7)\overline{4.00} \quad \leftarrow \text{Use 2 zeros}$$
$$\underline{0.5\ ⑦}$$

$$\therefore \frac{4}{7} \approx 0.6$$

[The symbol $\approx$ stands for *is approximately equal to*]

Example B

Change $\frac{5}{6}$ to a decimal correct to TWO decimal places

$$6)\overline{5.000} \quad \leftarrow \text{Use 3 zeros}$$
$$\underline{0.83\ ③}$$

$$\therefore \frac{5}{6} \approx 0.83$$

Example C

Change $\frac{13}{60}$ to a decimal correct to THREE decimal places

$$10)\overline{13.0}$$
$$6)\overline{1.3000} \quad \left[\begin{array}{l} \text{divide by 10} \\ \text{and then 6} \\ \text{since } 10 \times 6 = 60 \end{array} \right]$$
$$\underline{0.216\ ⑥}$$

$$\therefore \frac{13}{60} \approx 0.217$$

Exercise 1L

Part i   *Change each vulgar fraction to a decimal correct to ONE decimal place.*

1 $\frac{1}{3}$ 3 $\frac{2}{7}$ 5 $\frac{2}{9}$ 7 $\frac{6}{11}$

2 $\frac{5}{6}$ 4 $\frac{5}{7}$ 6 $\frac{3}{11}$ 8 $\frac{11}{12}$

Part ii   *Change each vulgar fraction to a decimal correct to TWO decimal places.*

1 $\frac{2}{3}$ 3 $\frac{6}{7}$ 5 $\frac{8}{9}$ 7 $\frac{10}{11}$

2 $\frac{1}{6}$ 4 $\frac{4}{9}$ 6 $\frac{4}{11}$ 8 $\frac{5}{12}$

Part iii   *Change each vulgar fraction to a decimal correct to THREE decimal places.*

1 $\frac{1}{30}$ 3 $\frac{7}{60}$ 5 $\frac{9}{70}$ 7 $\frac{1}{90}$

2 $\frac{17}{30}$ 4 $\frac{31}{60}$ 6 $\frac{53}{70}$ 8 $\frac{23}{90}$

Check your answers on p 126

VULGAR FRACTION TO A PERCENTAGE

Percentage means *parts in a hundred* or *parts per hundred*

Example A

Change $\dfrac{7}{20}$ to a percentage

$$\dfrac{7}{20} = \dfrac{7}{\cancel{20}_{1}} \times \dfrac{\overset{5}{\cancel{100}}}{1} \; \% \; [\text{'cancel' across by 20}]$$

$$= \dfrac{35}{1}\%$$

$$= 35\%$$

Example B

Change $\dfrac{3}{8}$ to a percentage

$$\dfrac{3}{8} = \dfrac{3}{\cancel{8}_{2}} \times \dfrac{\overset{25}{\cancel{100}}}{1} \; \% \; [\text{'cancel' across by 4}]$$

$$= \dfrac{75}{2}\%$$

$$= 37\tfrac{1}{2}\%$$

Exercise 1M   *Change to a percentage*

1 $\frac{1}{2}$

2 $\frac{1}{4}$

3 $\frac{3}{4}$

4 $\frac{1}{5}$

5 $\frac{2}{5}$

6 $\frac{3}{5}$

7 $\frac{4}{5}$

8 $\frac{1}{10}$

9 $\frac{3}{10}$

10 $\frac{7}{10}$

11 $\frac{9}{10}$

12 $\frac{1}{20}$

13 $\frac{3}{20}$

14 $\frac{9}{20}$

15 $\frac{11}{20}$

16 $\frac{13}{20}$

17 $\frac{17}{20}$

18 $\frac{19}{20}$

19 $\frac{1}{25}$

20 $\frac{3}{25}$

21 $\frac{7}{25}$

22 $\frac{11}{25}$

23 $\frac{13}{25}$

24 $\frac{17}{25}$

25 $\frac{19}{25}$

26 $\frac{23}{25}$

27 $\frac{1}{3}$

28 $\frac{2}{3}$

29 $\frac{1}{8}$

30 $\frac{5}{8}$

31 $\frac{7}{8}$

32 $\frac{1}{6}$

33 $\frac{5}{6}$

34 $\frac{1}{9}$

35 $\frac{4}{9}$

36 $\frac{7}{9}$

37 $\frac{1}{40}$

38 $\frac{3}{40}$

39 $\frac{9}{40}$

40 $\frac{11}{40}$

Check your answers on p 127

DILUTION RATIOS

The strength of a solution may be given as a ratio in either of two ways, e.g. '1 in 4' is equivalent to '1 to 3' (1 to 3 may be written as 1 : 3).

1 in 4 means 1 part of stock solution added *in* 4 parts of diluted solution.

1 : 3 means 1 part of stock solution added *to* 3 parts of diluent. (*Diluent: a substance that dilutes or dissolves.*)

Example A

Change the ratio 1 : 5 to the form 1 in x

   1 + 5 = 6 parts

∴ 1 : 5 = 1 in 6

Example B

Change the ratio 1 in 10 to the form 1 : y

   10 − 1 = 9 parts of diluent

∴ 1 in 10 = 1 : 9

Example C

How much stock solution is present in 200 mL of diluted solution if the strength of the solution is

a *1 in 5*

a 1 in 5 = $\frac{1}{5}$

$\frac{1}{5} \times 200$ mL = 40 mL

b *1 : 5?*

b 1 : 5 = 1 in 6 = $\frac{1}{6}$

$\frac{1}{6} \times 200$ mL = 33 mL (to the nearest mL)

Note

A ratio may be written as a fraction.

Exercise 1N

Part i   *Change these ratios to the form 1 in x.*

1 1 : 2	**4** 1 : 10	**7** 1 : 30	**10** 1 : 200
2 1 : 5	**5** 1 : 15	**8** 1 : 50	**11** 1 : 250
3 1 : 7	**6** 1 : 25	**9** 1 : 100	**12** 1 : 500

Part ii   *Change these ratios to the form 1 : y*

1 1 in 2	**4** 1 in 7	**7** 1 in 20	**10** 1 in 50
2 1 in 3	**5** 1 in 10	**8** 1 in 25	**11** 1 in 100
3 1 in 5	**6** 1 in 15	**9** 1 in 40	**12** 1 in 200

Part iii   *How much stock solution is present in the given volume of diluted solution? Calculate answers to the nearest millilitre.*

Volume of diluted solution	Dilution ratios a	b
1 100 mL	1 in 4	1 : 4
2 150 mL	1 in 2	1 : 2
3 300 mL	1 in 5	1 : 5
4 600 mL	1 in 3	1 : 3
5 420 mL	1 in 6	1 : 6
6 550 mL	1 in 10	1 : 10
7 400 mL	1 in 3	1 : 3
8 750 mL	1 in 4	1 : 4
9 900 mL	1 in 6	1 : 6
10 1 litre	1 in 7	1 : 7
11 2 litre	1 in 8	1 : 8
12 5 litre	1 in 9	1 : 9

Check your answers on p 127

RATIO TO A PERCENTAGE

The strength of a solution may be given as a ratio (e.g. 1 in 5 or 1 : 4) or as a percentage (20%).

Example A

Change the ratio 1 in 40 to a percentage

$$1 \text{ in } 40 = \frac{1}{\underset{2}{\cancel{40}}} \times \frac{\overset{5}{\cancel{100}}}{1} \% \text{ ['cancel' across by 20]}$$

$$= \frac{5}{2} \% \text{ or } 2.5\%$$

Example B

Change 1 in 500 to a percentage

$$1 \text{ in } 500 = \frac{1}{\underset{5}{\cancel{500}}} \times \frac{\overset{1}{\cancel{100}}}{1} \%$$

$$= \frac{1}{5} \% \text{ or } 0.2\% \text{ [note answer } less \text{ } than \text{ } 1\%]$$

$$5\overline{)\,1.000} \\ \quad\; 0.2$$

Example C

Change 1 in 600 to a percentage correct to 0.01%

$$1 \text{ in } 600 = \frac{1}{\underset{6}{\cancel{600}}} \times \frac{\overset{1}{\cancel{100}}}{1} \%$$

$$= \frac{1}{6} \% \approx 0.17\%$$

$$6\overline{)\,1.000} \\ \quad\; 0.16\,\textcircled{6}$$

Example D

Change 1 : 10 to a percentage correct to two decimal places

$$1 : 10 = 1 \text{ in } 11$$

$$= \frac{1}{11} \times \frac{100}{1} \%$$

$$= \frac{100}{11} \% \text{ or } 9.09\%$$

$$11\overline{)\,100.000} \\ \quad\;\; 9.09\,\textcircled{0}$$

Exercise 10   *Change each ratio to a percentage correct to two decimal places (where necessary).*

1 1 in 2	**17** 1 in 3	**33** 1 in 800
2 1 in 4	**18** 1 in 6	**34** 1 in 900
3 1 in 5	**19** 1 in 7	**35** *Can you see the*
4 1 in 10	**20** 1 in 8	*relationship between:*
5 1 in 20	**21** 1 in 9	*1 in 2, 1 in 20, 1 in 200;*
6 1 in 25	**22** 1 in 12	*or 1 in 3, 1 in 30, 1 in*
7 1 in 50	**23** 1 in 15	*300, etc...?*
8 1 in 100	**24** 1 in 30	
9 1 in 200	**25** 1 in 60	
10 1 in 250	**26** 1 in 70	*Now do these:*
11 1 in 400	**27** 1 in 75	**36** 1 : 2
12 1 in 1000	**28** 1 in 80	**37** 1 : 3
13 1 in 2000	**29** 1 in 90	**38** 1 : 5
14 1 in 2500	**30** 1 in 300	**39** 1 : 6
15 1 in 5000	**31** 1 in 400	**40** 1 : 7
16 1 in 10 000	**32** 1 in 700	**41** 1 : 8
		42 1 : 9

Note

A ratio may be written as a fraction or an equivalent percentage (e.g. 1 in 5 = $\frac{1}{5}$ = 20%).

Check your answers on p 128

DECIMAL FRACTION TO VULGAR FRACTION

Many syringes with a capacity of more than 1 mL are graduated in *tenths* of a millilitre.

$\frac{1}{10}$ mL = 0.01 mL

Syringes designed to hold 1 mL or less are often graduated in *hundredths* of a millilitre.

$\frac{1}{100}$ mL = 0.1 mL

Example A

Change 0.4 to a vulgar fraction and simplify

$$0.4 = \frac{4}{10}$$
$$= \frac{2}{5}$$

Example B

Change 0.36 to a vulgar fraction and simplify

$$0.36 = \frac{36}{100}$$
$$= \frac{9}{25}$$

Exercise 1P   *Change to a vulgar fraction and simplify where possible.*

Part i

1 0.1	**3** 0.3	**5** 0.6	**7** 0.8
2 0.2	**4** 0.5	**6** 0.7	**8** 0.9

Part ii

1 0.24	**11** 0.03	**21** 0.75	**31** 0.57
2 0.46	**12** 0.72	**22** 0.26	**32** 0.87
3 0.77	**13** 0.65	**23** 0.39	**33** 0.41
4 0.13	**14** 0.25	**24** 0.53	**34** 0.08
5 0.35	**15** 0.36	**25** 0.18	**35** 0.64
6 0.81	**16** 0.58	**26** 0.69	**36** 0.28
7 0.66	**17** 0.16	**27** 0.48	**37** 0.79
8 0.01	**18** 0.83	**28** 0.05	**38** 0.38
9 0.95	**19** 0.45	**29** 0.85	**39** 0.99
10 0.55	**20** 0.96	**30** 0.92	**40** 0.15

Check your answers on p 128–9

PERCENTAGE TO VULGAR FRACTION

The strength of a solution may be expressed as a percentage or as a ratio, e.g. 25% or 1 in 4 or 1 : 3. The ratio 1 in 4 can be written as a fraction $\frac{1}{4}$.

Example A   *Change 16% to a vulgar fraction*

$$16\% \ = \ \frac{16}{100}$$

$$= \ \frac{4}{25} \qquad \text{[always simplify if possible]}$$

Example B

i Change 0.3% to a vulgar fraction

$$0.3\% \ = \ \frac{0.3}{100} \quad \begin{bmatrix} \text{multiply numerator} \\ \text{and denominator by 10} \end{bmatrix}$$

$$= \ \frac{3}{1000} \quad \text{which cannot be simplified}$$

ii Change 0.08% to a vulgar fraction

$$0.08\% \ = \ \frac{0.08}{100} \quad \begin{bmatrix} \text{multiply numerator} \\ \text{and denominator by 100} \end{bmatrix}$$

$$= \ \frac{8}{10\,000}$$

$$= \ \frac{1}{1250}$$

Example C

Change $3\frac{1}{2}$ % to a vulgar fraction

$$3\frac{1}{2}\% \ = \ \frac{3\frac{1}{2}}{100} \quad \begin{bmatrix} \text{multiply numerator} \\ \text{and denominator by 2} \end{bmatrix}$$

$$= \ \frac{7}{200} \qquad \text{which cannot be simplified}$$

Exercise 1Q   *Change each percentage to a vulgar fraction and simplify ('cancel down') if possible.*

Part i

1 2%	**6** 10%	**11** 35%
2 3%	**7** 12%	**12** 40%
3 4%	**8** 15%	**13** 45%
4 5%	**9** 20%	**14** 50%
5 7%	**10** 30%	**15** 90%

Part ii

1 0.1%	**6** 0.7%	**11** 0.04%
2 0.2%	**7** 0.8%	**12** 0.05%
3 0.4%	**8** 0.9%	**13** 0.06%
4 0.5%	**9** 0.01%	**14** 0.07%
5 0.6%	**10** 0.02%	**15** 0.09%

Part iii

1 $\frac{1}{2}$ %	**3** $2\frac{1}{2}$ %	**5** $7\frac{1}{2}$ %
2 $1\frac{1}{2}$ %	**4** $4\frac{1}{2}$ %	**6** $12\frac{1}{2}$ %

Note
A percentage may be changed to a fraction or an equivalent ratio (e.g. 5% = $\frac{1}{20}$ = 1 in 20).

Check your answers on p 129

MIXED NUMBERS AND IMPROPER FRACTIONS

Example A

i Change $\dfrac{17}{5}$ to a mixed number

$$\dfrac{17}{5} = 17 \div 5$$

$$= 3\dfrac{2}{5} \quad \begin{array}{l} \leftarrow \text{remainder} \\ \leftarrow \text{same denominator as improper fraction} \end{array} \Big]$$

ii Change $\dfrac{115}{4}$ to a mixed number

$$\dfrac{115}{4} = 115 \div 4$$

$$= 28\dfrac{3}{4} \quad \begin{array}{l} \leftarrow \text{remainder} \\ \leftarrow \text{same denominator as improper fraction} \end{array} \Big]$$

Example B

i Change $8\dfrac{1}{4}$ to an improper fraction

$$8\dfrac{1}{4} = \dfrac{33}{4} \quad \begin{array}{l} \leftarrow 8 \times 4 + 1 \\ \leftarrow \text{same denominator as fraction in mixed number} \end{array} \Big]$$

ii Change $20\dfrac{4}{5}$ to an improper fraction

$$20\dfrac{4}{5} = \dfrac{104}{5} \quad \begin{array}{l} \leftarrow 20 \times 5 + 4 \\ \leftarrow \text{same denominator as fraction in mixed number} \end{array} \Big]$$

Exercise 1R

Part i *Change these improper fractions to mixed numbers.*

1 $\frac{5}{2}$ 5 $\frac{29}{6}$ 9 $\frac{51}{2}$ 13 $\frac{95}{6}$ 17 $\frac{133}{5}$

2 $\frac{11}{3}$ 6 $\frac{36}{7}$ 10 $\frac{65}{3}$ 14 $\frac{101}{7}$ 18 $\frac{143}{6}$

3 $\frac{17}{4}$ 7 $\frac{37}{8}$ 11 $\frac{71}{4}$ 15 $\frac{113}{8}$ 19 $\frac{157}{7}$

4 $\frac{22}{5}$ 8 $\frac{49}{9}$ 12 $\frac{86}{5}$ 16 $\frac{125}{9}$ 20 $\frac{166}{9}$

Part ii *Rewrite these mixed numbers as improper fractions.*

1 $1\frac{1}{2}$ 5 $3\frac{1}{2}$ 9 $11\frac{1}{6}$ 13 $22\frac{1}{2}$ 17 $30\frac{5}{6}$

2 $1\frac{1}{3}$ 6 $4\frac{2}{3}$ 10 $13\frac{2}{7}$ 14 $24\frac{2}{3}$ 18 $32\frac{4}{7}$

3 $1\frac{3}{4}$ 7 $6\frac{1}{4}$ 11 $16\frac{5}{8}$ 15 $27\frac{3}{4}$ 19 $35\frac{3}{8}$

4 $2\frac{3}{5}$ 8 $9\frac{4}{5}$ 12 $17\frac{2}{9}$ 16 $29\frac{1}{5}$ 20 $38\frac{5}{9}$

Check your answers on p 130

MULTIPLICATION OF VULGAR FRACTIONS

Example A $\dfrac{2}{5} \times \dfrac{4}{7}$

$$\dfrac{2}{5} \times \dfrac{4}{7} = \dfrac{2 \times 4}{5 \times 7}$$

$$= \dfrac{8}{35} \quad \left[\begin{array}{l}\text{this fraction can}\\\text{not be simplified}\end{array}\right]$$

Example B $\dfrac{5}{8} \times \dfrac{7}{10}$

$$\dfrac{\overset{1}{\cancel{5}}}{8} \times \dfrac{7}{\underset{2}{\cancel{10}}} = \dfrac{1 \times 7}{8 \times 2} \quad \left[\begin{array}{l}\text{note cancelling}\\\text{across by 5}\end{array}\right]$$

$$= \dfrac{7}{16}$$

Example C $\dfrac{4}{9} \times \dfrac{21}{5}$

$$\dfrac{4}{\underset{3}{\cancel{9}}} \times \dfrac{\overset{7}{\cancel{21}}}{5} = \dfrac{4 \times 7}{3 \times 5} \quad \left[\begin{array}{l}\text{note cancelling}\\\text{across by 3}\end{array}\right]$$

$$= \dfrac{28}{15}$$

$$= 1\tfrac{13}{15} \quad \text{[answers may be greater than one]}$$

Example D $\dfrac{9}{10} \times \dfrac{8}{15}$

$$\dfrac{\overset{3}{\cancel{9}}}{\underset{5}{\cancel{10}}} \times \dfrac{\overset{4}{\cancel{8}}}{\underset{5}{\cancel{15}}} = \dfrac{3 \times 4}{5 \times 5} \quad \left[\begin{array}{l}\text{note cancelling across}\\\text{by 3 and by 2}\end{array}\right]$$

$$= \dfrac{12}{25}$$

Exercise 1S   *Multiply. Simplify where possible.*

1 $\dfrac{1}{2} \times \dfrac{2}{5}$

2 $\dfrac{1}{3} \times \dfrac{5}{8}$

3 $\dfrac{2}{3} \times \dfrac{5}{6}$

4 $\dfrac{1}{4} \times \dfrac{2}{3}$

5 $\dfrac{3}{4} \times \dfrac{20}{9}$

6 $\dfrac{1}{5} \times \dfrac{3}{10}$

7 $\dfrac{2}{5} \times \dfrac{3}{2}$

8 $\dfrac{3}{5} \times \dfrac{3}{4}$

9 $\dfrac{4}{5} \times \dfrac{25}{24}$

10 $\dfrac{1}{6} \times \dfrac{9}{10}$

11 $\dfrac{5}{6} \times \dfrac{8}{15}$

12 $\dfrac{1}{7} \times \dfrac{7}{18}$

13 $\dfrac{2}{7} \times \dfrac{11}{12}$

14 $\dfrac{3}{7} \times \dfrac{1}{20}$

15 $\dfrac{4}{7} \times \dfrac{5}{3}$

16 $\dfrac{5}{7} \times \dfrac{12}{25}$

17 $\dfrac{6}{7} \times \dfrac{5}{24}$

18 $\dfrac{1}{8} \times \dfrac{1}{2}$

19 $\dfrac{3}{8} \times \dfrac{12}{5}$

20 $\dfrac{5}{8} \times \dfrac{9}{20}$

21 $\dfrac{7}{8} \times \dfrac{8}{7}$

22 $\dfrac{1}{9} \times \dfrac{1}{15}$

23 $\dfrac{2}{9} \times \dfrac{7}{4}$

24 $\dfrac{4}{9} \times \dfrac{5}{12}$

25 $\dfrac{5}{9} \times \dfrac{21}{25}$

26 $\dfrac{7}{9} \times \dfrac{9}{16}$

27 $\dfrac{8}{9} \times \dfrac{1}{6}$

28 $\dfrac{1}{10} \times \dfrac{15}{8}$

29 $\dfrac{3}{10} \times \dfrac{4}{9}$

30 $\dfrac{7}{10} \times \dfrac{2}{7}$

31 $\dfrac{9}{10} \times \dfrac{15}{16}$

32 $\dfrac{1}{11} \times \dfrac{11}{18}$

33 $\dfrac{1}{12} \times \dfrac{1}{30}$

34 $\dfrac{5}{12} \times \dfrac{7}{30}$

35 $\dfrac{7}{12} \times \dfrac{9}{40}$

36 $\dfrac{11}{12} \times \dfrac{33}{40}$

Check your answers on p 130

DIVISION BY A VULGAR FRACTION

Drug dosage and dilution calculations often involve division by a vulgar fraction.

Method
To divide by a vulgar fraction, invert the divisor and then multiply.
(*Note:* the *divisor* is the number you are dividing by.)
or
To divide by a vulgar fraction, multiply by its reciprocal.

(*Note:* the *reciprocal* of $\frac{a}{b}$ is $\frac{b}{a}$)

Example A $\quad \dfrac{2}{3} \div \dfrac{4}{5}$

$$\frac{2}{3} \div \frac{4}{5} = \frac{\overset{1}{\cancel{2}}}{3} \times \frac{5}{\underset{2}{\cancel{4}}} \qquad [\text{'cancelling' across by 2}]$$

$$= \frac{5}{6}$$

Example B $\quad \dfrac{9}{10} \div \dfrac{6}{7}$

$$\frac{9}{10} \div \frac{6}{7} = \frac{\overset{3}{\cancel{9}}}{10} \times \frac{7}{\underset{2}{\cancel{6}}} \qquad [\text{'cancelling' across by 3}]$$

$$= \frac{21}{20}$$

$$= 1\frac{1}{20}$$

Exercise 1T   *Divide. Simplify where possible.*

1 $\frac{1}{2} \div \frac{3}{4}$ **13** $\frac{3}{5} \div \frac{9}{10}$ **25** $\frac{5}{8} \div \frac{5}{6}$

2 $\frac{1}{2} \div \frac{1}{3}$ **14** $\frac{4}{5} \div \frac{2}{3}$ **26** $\frac{7}{8} \div \frac{1}{2}$

3 $\frac{1}{3} \div \frac{1}{4}$ **15** $\frac{1}{6} \div \frac{7}{9}$ **27** $\frac{1}{9} \div \frac{1}{5}$

4 $\frac{1}{3} \div \frac{5}{9}$ **16** $\frac{5}{6} \div \frac{2}{5}$ **28** $\frac{2}{9} \div \frac{2}{3}$

5 $\frac{2}{3} \div \frac{1}{6}$ **17** $\frac{1}{7} \div \frac{1}{8}$ **29** $\frac{4}{9} \div \frac{1}{6}$

6 $\frac{2}{3} \div \frac{4}{9}$ **18** $\frac{2}{7} \div \frac{4}{5}$ **30** $\frac{5}{9} \div \frac{5}{8}$

7 $\frac{1}{4} \div \frac{1}{2}$ **19** $\frac{3}{7} \div \frac{9}{10}$ **31** $\frac{7}{9} \div \frac{7}{10}$

8 $\frac{1}{4} \div \frac{4}{5}$ **20** $\frac{4}{7} \div \frac{1}{3}$ **32** $\frac{8}{9} \div \frac{2}{3}$

9 $\frac{3}{4} \div \frac{5}{6}$ **21** $\frac{5}{7} \div \frac{10}{3}$ **33** $\frac{1}{10} \div \frac{1}{7}$

10 $\frac{3}{4} \div \frac{1}{5}$ **22** $\frac{6}{7} \div \frac{3}{4}$ **34** $\frac{3}{10} \div \frac{5}{6}$

11 $\frac{1}{5} \div \frac{1}{3}$ **23** $\frac{1}{8} \div \frac{7}{8}$ **35** $\frac{7}{10} \div \frac{7}{8}$

12 $\frac{2}{5} \div \frac{3}{5}$ **24** $\frac{3}{8} \div \frac{9}{10}$ **36** $\frac{9}{10} \div \frac{3}{5}$

Check your answers on p 131

2. Drug dosages for injection

Correct measurement of drug dosages for injection is most important. An overdose can be dangerous; too low a dose may result in a drug being ineffective.

The number of decimal places in each answer should match the graduations on the syringe being used. Syringes with a capacity of more than 1 mL are usually graduated in tenths or fifths of a mL: so for volumes *greater* than 1 mL calculate answers correct to *one* decimal place. Syringes with a capacity of 1 mL or less are often graduated in hundredths of a mL: so for volumes *less* than 1 mL calculate answers to *two* decimal places.

Check that stock strength and the strength required are given in the *same* unit in a particular problem (i.e. *both* strengths in grams or milligrams or micrograms).

Be **very careful** when working in **micrograms** — write the word 'micrograms' in full rather than the Greek μ, to avoid any confusion.

Important: if in *any* doubt about the answer to a calculation, ask a supervisor to *check* your calculation.

Example 1 *Pethidine 75 mg is to be given I.M.I. Stock ampoules of pethidine contain 100 mg in 2 mL. Is the volume to be drawn up for injection equal to 2 mL, less than 2 mL, or more than 2 mL?*

A stock ampoule contains 100 mg of pethidine.
Volume of ampoule = 2 mL
75 mg (prescribed) is *less than* 100 mg (ampoule).
Therefore, volume to be drawn up is *less than* 2 mL.

Example 2 *Methicillin 1800 mg is ordered. Stock ampoules contain 1 g/3 mL. Is the volume of stock required for injection equal to 3 mL, less than 3 mL, or more than 3 mL?*

A stock ampoule contains 1 g of methicillin.
1 g = 1 gram = 1000 mg
Volume of ampoule = 3 mL
1800 mg (prescribed) is *more than* 1000 mg (ampoule).
Therefore, volume required is *more than* 3 mL.

Example 3 *A patient is to be given 12 000 units of Calciparine. Available ampoules contain 25 000 U in 1 mL. Should the volume to be drawn up for injection be equal to 1 mL, less than 1 mL, or more than 1 mL?*

A stock ampoule contains 25 000 U [U for units].
Volume of ampoule = 1 mL
12 000 units (prescribed) is *less than* 25 000 units (ampoule).
Therefore, volume to be drawn up is *less than* 1 mL.

Exercise 2A

Rewrite the correct answer to each problem. The answer will be either equal to, less than, or more than the volume of the stock ampoule.

1 An injection of morphine 9 mg is ordered. A stock ampoule contains morphine 15 mg in 1 mL. The volume to be drawn up for injection will be equal to 1 mL/less than 1 mL/more than 1 mL.

2 A patient is to receive an injection of erythromycin 170 mg. Stock vials contain erythromycin 100 mg/2 mL. The volume to be drawn up for injection is equal to 2 mL/less than 2 mL/more than 2 mL.

3 Cortisone 80 mg is ordered. Ampoules contain cortisone 125 mg in 5 mL. The volume required for injection is equal to 5 mL/less than 5 mL/more than 5 mL.

4 Penicillin 450 000 units is ordered. Stock ampoules contain 1 million units in 2 mL. The volume of stock required is equal to 2 mL/less than 2 mL/more than 2 mL.

5 A patient is prescribed capreomycin sulphate 1000 mg, I.M.I. If stock ampoules contain 1 gram in 3 mL, then the amount of stock solution to be drawn up will be equal to 3 mL/less than 3 mL/more than 3 mL.

6 On hand are digoxin ampoules containing 500 mg in 2 mL. An injection of digoxin 225 mg is ordered. The volume required is equal to 2 mL/less than 2 mL/more than 2 mL.

7 Heparin is available at a strength of 1000 units per mL. The volume needed to give 1250 units is equal to 1 mL/less than 1 mL/more than 1 mL.

Think carefully about each answer in the exercises which follow. Should the volume to be drawn up for injection be equal to, less than, or more than the volume of the stock ampoule?

Check your answers on p 131

Example 4   *A patient is ordered cortisone 40 mg, I.M.I. Ampoules contain cortisone 50 mg in 2 mL. Calculate the volume required for injection.*

$$\text{Volume required} = \frac{\text{Strength required}}{\text{Stock strength}} \times \left[\begin{array}{c} \text{Volume of} \\ \text{stock solution} \end{array} \right]$$

$$= \frac{40 \text{ mg}}{50 \text{ mg}} \times 2 \text{ mL}$$

$$= \frac{40}{50} \times \frac{2}{1} \text{ mL}$$

$$= \frac{8}{5} \text{ mL or 1.6 mL}$$

Example 5   *An injection of digoxin 175 microgram is ordered. Stock on hand is digoxin 500 microgram in 2 mL. What volume of stock solution should be given? (N.B. micrograms)*

$$\text{Volume required} = \frac{\text{Strength required}}{\text{Stock strength}} \times \left[\begin{array}{c} \text{Volume of} \\ \text{stock solution} \end{array} \right]$$

$$= \frac{175 \text{ microgram}}{500 \text{ microgram}} \times 2 \text{ mL}$$

$$= \frac{175}{500} \times \frac{2}{1} \text{ mL}$$

$$= \frac{7}{10} \text{ mL or 0.7 mL}$$

Exercise 2B

Stock strength refers to the strength of the medication supplied.

1 An injection of morphine 8 mg is required. Ampoules on hand contain 10 mg in 1 mL. What volume is drawn up for injection?

2 Digoxin ampoules on hand contain 500 microgram in 2 mL. What volume is needed to give 350 microgram?

3 A child is ordered 9 mg of gentamicin by I.M.I. Stock ampoules contain 20 mg in 2 mL. What volume is needed for the injection?

4 A patient is to be given erythromycin 120 mg by injection. Stock vials contain 300 mg/10 mL. Calculate the required volume.

5 Stock heparin has a strength of 5000 units per mL. What volume must be drawn up to give 6500 units?

6 Pethidine 85 mg is to be given I.M. Stock ampoules contain pethidine 100 mg in 2 mL. Calculate volume of stock required.

7 A patient is to receive an injection of gentamicin 60 mg, I.M. Ampoules on hand contain 80 mg/2 mL. Calculate volume required.

8 A patient is prescribed bumetanide 0.8 mg, I.M.I. Stock ampoules contain 2 mg/4 mL. What volume should be drawn up for injection?

Think about each answer. Does it make sense? Is it ridiculously large?

Check your answers on p 131

Exercise 2C

1 Kanamycin 500 mg is ordered. Stock on hand contains 1 gram in 3 mL. What volume is required?

2 A patient is to receive an injection of erythromycin 160 mg. Stock ampoules contain 100 mg in 2 mL. Calculate the volume to be drawn up for injection.

3 How much morphine solution must be withdrawn for a 7.5 mg dose if a stock ampoule contains 15 mg in 1 mL?

4 A patient is ordered 2 megaunits of crystalline penicillin. Stock is 5 megaunits in 10 mL. Calculate the volume that is needed.

5 Heparin is available at a strength of 5000 units/5 mL. What volume is needed to give 800 units?

6 Phenobarbitone 40 mg has been ordered. Stock ampoules contain 200 mg/mL. What volume should be given?

7 A patient is ordered pethidine 65 mg. Stock ampoules of pethidine contain 100 mg in 2 mL. Calculate the volume to de drawn up for injection.

8 A patient is to be given ranitidine 40 mg, I.V. Stock ampoules have a strength of 50 mg/2 mL. What volume of stock should be injected?

9 Apomorphine 5.5 mg is prescribed. Stock ampoules contain 10 mg/mL. What volume should be drawn up for injection?

Check your answers on p 131

Exercise 2D   *Calculate the volume of stock to be drawn up for injection.*

1   A patient is prescribed erythromycin 80 mg by I.M.I. Stock ampoules contain 100 mg/2 mL.

2   Pethidine 60 mg is ordered. Stock ampoules contain 100 mg in 2 mL.

3   An adult is ordered Omnopon 15 mg, premedication. On hand are ampoules containing 20 mg/mL.

4   A patient is ordered benzathine penicillin 150 000 units. On hand is benzathine penicillin 1.2 megaunits in 2 mL.

5   Cortisone 60 mg is required. Available stock contains 125 mg in 5 mL.

6   An adult patient with TB is to be given 500 mg of capreomycin sulphate every second day, I.M.I. Stock ampoules contain 1 gram in 3 mL.

7   Digoxin ampoules on hand contain 500 microgram in 2 mL. Digoxin 150 microgram is ordered.

8   Stock Calciparine contains 25 000 units in 1 mL. 15 000 units of Calciparine are ordered.

9   Penicillin 400 000 units is ordered. Stock ampoules contain 1 megaunit in 2 mL.

Note
1 megaunit = 1 million units. The symbol for megaunit is Mu.

Check your answers on p 132

Exercise 2E *Calculate the amount of stock solution to be drawn up for injection. Give answers greater than 1 mL correct to one decimal place; answers less than 1 mL correct to 2 decimal places. If the next decimal place is 5 or more, add one to the previous digit.*

1 Ordered : erythromycin 200 mg
   Stock   : 300 mg in 10 mL

2 Ordered : morphine 20 mg
   Stock   : 15 mg in 1 mL

3 Ordered : atropine 0.5 mg
   Stock   : 0.6 mg in 1 mL

4 Ordered : atropine 800 microgram
   Stock   : 1.2 mg in 1 mL

5 Ordered : benzathine penicillin 400 000 units
   Stock   : 1.2 Mu/2 mL

6 Ordered : capreomycin sulphate 850 mg
   Stock   : 2 grams per mL

7 Ordered : metoclopramide 7 mg
   Stock   : 10 mg/2 mL

8 Ordered : heparin 1750 units
   Stock   : 1000 units per mL

9 Ordered : scopolamine 0.25 mg
   Stock   : 0.4 mg/2 mL

Check your answers on p 132

Exercise 2F *Calculate the volume of stock required.*

	Ordered		Stock ampoule
1	Morphine	12 mg	15 mg/mL
2	Calciparine	7000 units	25 000 U in 1 mL
3	Crystalline penicillin	3.5 megaunits	5 megaunits in 10 mL
4	Heparin	3000 units	5000 U/mL
5	Phenobarbitone	70 mg	200 mg/mL
6	Pethidine	80 mg	100 mg/2 mL
7	Scopolamine	0.24 mg	0.4 mg/2 mL
8	Digoxin	200 microgram	500 microgram in 2 mL
9	Cortisone	75 mg	125 mg in 5 mL
10	Cortisone	90 mg	250 mg in 10 mL
11	Capreomycin sulphate	800 mg	1 gram in 5 mL
12	Crystalline penicillin	150 000 units	1 million units in 2 mL
13	Chloramphenicol	75 mg	250 mg in 5 mL
14	Methicillin	1500 mg	1 gram in 5 mL
15	Morphine	7.5 mg	10 mg in 1 mL
16	Methicillin	2100 mg	1 g/3 mL
17	Omnopon	34 mg	20 mg in 1 mL
18	Dexamethasone	3 mg	4 mg/mL
19	Benzathine penicillin	900 000 U	1.2 Mu/2 mL
20	Chlorpromazine	18 mg	25 mg/mL

Check your answers on p 132

Excercise 2G *The drawings represent syringes (needles not shown).*
For each pair of syringes, write down the volume (or units) of solution

  i between adjacent graduations
 ii indicated by arrow A
iii indicated by arrow B

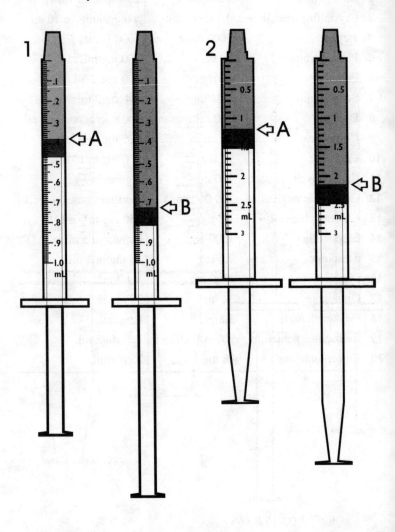

Note that syringes 3A and 3B are graduated in **units**, especially for **insulin** injections.

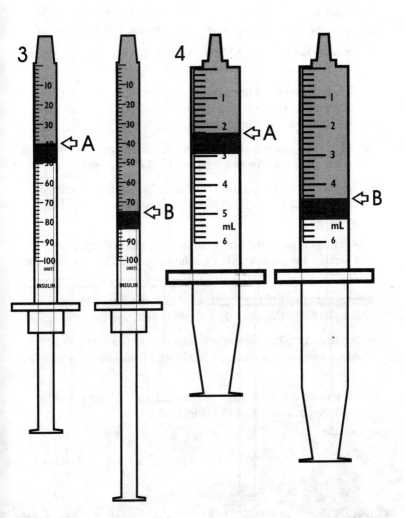

Check your answers on p 132

CHAPTER 2   Revision

1 Phenobarbitone 60 mg is to be given I.M.I. Stock ampoules contain 200 mg/mL. Is the volume of stock required equal to 1 mL, less than 1 mL, or more than 1 mL?

2 Pethidine 70 mg is to be given I.M.I. Calculate the volume of stock required if ampoules contain pethidine 100 mg in 2 mL.

3 Heparin 12 000 units, I.M.I. is ordered. Stock ampoules contain 25 000 U/5 mL. What volume should be drawn up?

4 A patient is ordered benzathine penicillin 240 000 units. On hand is benzathine penicillin 1.2 megaunits in 2 mL. Calculate the volume to be drawn up for injection.

5 Digoxin ampoules on hand contain 500 microgram in 2 mL. What volume is needed for an injection of 275 microgram?

6 A patient is ordered cortisone 70 mg, I.M.I. Ampoules contain cortisone 125 mg in 5 mL. Calculate the volume required for injection.

7 A patient is prescribed capreomycin sulphate 900 mg, I.M.I. Calculate the amount of stock solution required if stock ampoules contain 2 gram per mL.

8 Scopolamine 0.18 mg is ordered. Stock ampoules contain 0.4 mg/2 mL. Calculate the volume to be drawn up for injection.

9 A patient is to be given an injection of erythromycin 190 mg. Stock ampoules contain 300 mg/10 mL. Calculate the required volume.

10 How much morphine must be drawn up for a 10 mg dose if a stock ampoule contains 15 mg in 1 mL?

Check your answers on p 133

3. Dosages of tablets and mixtures

Drugs may be administered by injection, by I.V. infusion, or orally. Oral dosages may be in the form of tablets, capsules or mixtures.

Whole tablets are *always* preferable to broken tablets. Tablets of penicillin or other antibiotics should *never* be broken.

For other drugs, never use less than half a tablet. If a tablet *has* to be broken into 'halves' then use the other 'half' of the tablet for the next dose.

Many mixtures are *suspensions*. These must be shaken thoroughly, in order to obtain the correct stock strength, before measuring out the required volume.

Example 1 *How many 30 mg tablets of phenobarbitone should be given for a dose of phenobarbitone 45 mg?*

$$\text{Volume required} = \frac{\text{Strength required}}{\text{Stock strength}} \times \left[\begin{array}{c} \text{Volume of} \\ \text{stock solution} \end{array} \right]$$

$$= \frac{45 \text{ mg}}{30 \text{ mg}} \times 1 \text{ tablet}$$

$$= 1\tfrac{1}{2} \text{ tablets}$$

Example 2 *A patient is ordered 0.25 mg of digoxin, orally. The digoxin available is in tablets containing 125 microgram. How many such tablets should the patient receive?*

Change both strengths to the same unit

$$0.25 \text{ mg} = 250 \text{ microgram}$$

$$\therefore \text{Volume required} = \frac{\text{Strength required}}{\text{Stock strength}} \times \left[\begin{array}{c} \text{Volume of} \\ \text{stock solution} \end{array} \right]$$

$$= \frac{250 \text{ microgram}}{125 \text{ microgram}} \times 1 \text{ tablet}$$

$$= 2 \text{ tablets}$$

Note

In the case of tablets, 'volume required' refers to the number of tablets.

Exercise 3A

1 A patient is ordered penicillin 375 mg, orally. Stock on hand is 125 mg tablets. Calculate the number of tablets required.

2 How many 30 mg tablets of codeine are needed for a dose of 0.06 gram?

3 A patient is ordered ranitidine 225 mg, orally. In the ward are 150 mg tablets. How many tablets should be given?

4 Ordered: codeine 15 mg, orally. Stock on hand: codeine tablets, 30 mg. How many tablets should the patient take?

5 750 mg of penicillin is required. On hand are tablets of strength 250 mg. How many tablets should be given?

6 A patient is prescribed 150 mg of soluble aspirin. On hand are 300 mg tablets. What number should be given?

7 450 mg of soluble aspirin is ordered. Stock on hand is 300 mg tablets. How many tablets should the patient receive?

8 25 mg of captopril is prescribed. How many 50 mg tablets should be given?

*Check that you have used the **same unit of weight** throughout a calculation. Are **both** weights in milligram (mg)? Or are **both** weights in microgram?*

Check your answers on p 133

For some medications, tablets are available in different strengths. The tablets are colour-coded to reduce the risk of error when dispensing.

Example 3 *Choose the best combination of 1 mg, 2 mg, 5 mg or 10 mg tablets of warfarin for each of these dosages: i 6 mg ii 8 mg   iii 11 mg   iv 14 mg. The number of tablets should be as few as possible and only whole tablets may be used.*

i   5 mg + 1 mg (2 tabs)

ii   5 mg + 2 mg + 1 mg (3 tabs)

iii   10 mg + 1 mg (2 tabs)

iv   10 mg + 2 mg + 2 mg (3 tabs)

Exercise 3B *Choose the best combination of tablets for each of the following prescriptions. The **number** of tablets should be as few as possible and only **whole** tablets may be used.*

1 *Prescribed*: warfarin tablets
   Strengths available: 1 mg, 2 mg, 5 mg, 10 mg
   Dosages required: **a** 4 mg **b** 9 mg **c** 12 mg **d** 15 mg

2 *Prescribed*: diazepam tablets
   Strengths available: 2 mg, 5 mg, 10 mg
   Dosages required: **a** 7 mg **b** 9 mg **c** 15 mg **d** 20 mg

3 *Prescribed*: verapamil tablets
   Strengths available: 40 mg, 80 mg, 120 mg, 160 mg
   Dosages required: **a** 200 mg **b** 240 mg **c** 280 mg **d** 320 mg

4 *Prescribed*: prazosin tablets
   Strengths available: 1 mg, 2 mg, 5 mg
   Dosages required: **a** 6 mg **b** 8 mg **c** 9 mg **d** 11 mg

5 *Prescribed*: bromazepam tablets
   Strengths available: 3 mg, 6 mg, 12 mg
   Dosages required: **a** 9 mg **b** 15 mg **c** 18 mg **d** 21 mg

6 *Prescribed*: thioridazine tablets
   Strengths available: 10 mg, 25 mg, 50 mg, 100 mg
   Dosages required: **a** 35 mg **b** 60 mg **c** 75 mg **d** 120 mg

Check your answers on p 133–4

Example 4 *750 mg of erythromycin is to be given orally as a sedative. Stock suspension contains 250 mg/5 mL. Calculate the volume of mixture to be given.*

$$\begin{aligned}
\text{Volume} \atop \text{required} &= \frac{\text{Strength required}}{\text{Stock strength}} \times \left[\begin{array}{c} \text{Volume of} \\ \text{stock solution} \end{array} \right] \\[2mm]
&= \frac{750 \text{ mg}}{250 \text{ mg}} \times 5 \text{ mL} \\[2mm]
&= \frac{750}{250} \times \frac{5}{1} \text{ mL} \\[2mm]
&= 15 \text{ mL}
\end{aligned}$$

Example 5 *A patient is ordered 800 mg of penicillin, orally. Stock mixture on hand has a strength of 250 mg/5 mL. Calculate the volume required.*

$$\begin{aligned}
\text{Volume} \atop \text{required} &= \frac{\text{Strength required}}{\text{Stock strength}} \times \left[\begin{array}{c} \text{Volume of} \\ \text{stock solution} \end{array} \right] \\[2mm]
&= \frac{800 \text{ mg}}{250 \text{ mg}} \times 5 \text{ mL} \\[2mm]
&= \frac{800}{250} \times \frac{5}{1} \text{ mL} \\[2mm]
&= 16 \text{ mL}
\end{aligned}$$

Exercise 3C   *In each example, you are given the prescribed dosage and the strength of stock mixture on hand. Calculate the volume to be given.*

1 Ordered : penicillin 500 mg
   On hand : syrup 125 mg/5 mL

2 Ordered : aspirin 600 mg
   On hand : mixture 150 mg in 5 mL

3 Ordered : chloramphenicol 750 mg
   On hand : suspension 125 mg/5 mL

4 Ordered : sulphadiazine 2 gram
   On hand : mixture 500 mg/5 mL

5 Ordered : erythromycin 1250 mg
   On hand : suspension 250 mg/5 mL

6 Ordered : aspirin 900 mg
   On hand : mixture 150 mg in 5 mL

7 Ordered : penicillin 1000 mg
   On hand : mixture 250 mg/5 mL

8 Ordered : chlorpromazine 35 mg
   On hand : syrup 25 mg/5 mL

9 Ordered : penicillin 1200 mg
   On hand : mixture 250 mg/5 mL

10 Ordered : erythromycin 800 mg
    On hand : mixture 125 mg/5 mL

Check your answers on p 134

CHAPTER 3   **Revision**

1   A patient is ordered penicillin 500 mg orally. In the ward are 250 mg tablets. What number should be given?

2   12.5 mg of captopril is prescribed for hypertension. On hand are tablets of strength 25 mg. How many tablets should be given?

3   How many 30 mg tablets of codeine should be given for a dose of codeine 45 mg?

4   Choose the best combination of 1 mg, 2 mg, 5 mg and 10 mg tablets of warfarin for each of these dosages:
   a 3 mg   b 7 mg   c 13 mg   d 16 mg

5   Many mixtures are suspensions. What must be done to these mixtures before measuring out the required volume?

6   A patient is ordered 750 mg of erythromycin, orally. Calculate the volume required if the suspension on hand has a strength of 250 mg/5 mL.

7   Aspirin 750 mg is to be given as a mixture. Stock mixture contains 150 mg in 5 mL. Calculate the volume of mixture to be given.

8   A patient is prescribed penicillin 400 mg, orally. Stock syrup has a strength of 125 mg/5 mL. What volume should be given?

9   Flucloxacillin 375 mg is ordered. Stock syrup contains 125 mg/5 mL. What volume of syrup should the patient be given?

Check your answers on p 134

4. Dilution and strengths of solutions

Most solutions are stored in concentrated form in order to save storage space. The concentrated solution is then diluted before use. In most major hospitals, the diluting is done by pharmacy staff. However, in smaller hospitals, a nurse may have this responsibility.

The same substance may be used at different strengths for different purposes.

Strengths of solutions may be stated in grams per litre, mg/mL, as ratio strengths, or as percentage strengths. Every ratio strength has an equivalent percentage strength, and vice versa.

For *weak* (or very dilute) solutions, ratios such as

1 : 1000, 1 : 2000 and 1 : 5000 may be written as $\frac{1}{1000}$, $\frac{1}{2000}$ and $\frac{1}{5000}$ rather than $\frac{1}{1001}$, $\frac{1}{2001}$ and $\frac{1}{5001}$.

For *weak* solutions, this is sufficiently accurate for practical purposes.

Remember:
Percentage means parts per hundred parts.
e.g. 3% = 3 parts per hundred parts

$$= \frac{3}{100} \text{ (or 3 in 100).}$$

Example 1 *Calculate the percentage strength when 2 mL of disinfectant concentrate is made up to one litre with water.*

$$\text{One litre} = 1000 \text{ mL}$$

$$\text{Ratio strength} = \frac{2 \text{ mL}}{1000 \text{ mL}} = \frac{2}{1000}$$

$$\therefore \text{ Percentage strength} = \frac{2}{1000} \times \frac{100}{1} \% = 0.2\%$$

Example 2 *A 2.5% sodium hypochlorite solution is to be used to bathe a wound. Express 2.5% as a ratio strength.*

$$2.5\% = \frac{2.5}{100} \left[\begin{array}{l} \text{multiply numerator} \\ \text{and denominator by 10} \end{array} \right]$$

$$= \frac{25}{1000}$$

$$= \frac{1}{40} \text{ (or 1 in 40)}$$

Example 3 *Calculate the percentage strength of the solution when 10 g of silver nitrate is dissolved in 200 mL of water.*

200 mL of water weighs 200 gram

$$\text{Ratio strength} = \frac{10 \text{ g}}{200 \text{ g}} = \frac{10}{200}$$

$$\therefore \text{ Percentage strength} = \frac{10}{200} \times \frac{100}{1} \% = 5\%$$

*Note: This is not strictly correct as the 10 g of silver nitrate makes the weight of the **solution** 210 gram. However, the method is sufficiently accurate for practical purposes, and is used when a **solid** is dissolved in a liquid.*

Exercise 4A

1 Find the ratio strength of a solution when **a** 2 mL **b** 20 mL
   c 200 mL of pure substance is made up to 2 litre with water.

2 Change the following percentage strengths to ratio
   strengths:
   a 50% **b** 25% **c** 20% **d** 10% **e** 5%
   f $2\frac{1}{2}$% **g** 2% **h** 0.5% **i** 0.2% **j** 0.1%

3 Find (a) the ratio strength (b) the percentage strength of a solution
   after 15 mL of pure substance is mixed with 360 mL of water.

4 Find (a) the ratio strength (b) the percentage strength of the
   solution when 10 mL of concentrated disinfectant is made up to
   200 mL with water.

5 A sodium hypochlorite solution (Milton) has a strength of 1 in 80.
   Express this as a percentage strength.

6 Chlorhexidine is used as a 1 : 2000 solution for a general
   antiseptic; 1 : 5000 for douches. Change
   (a) 1 : 2000   (b) 1 : 5000 to percentages.

Check your answers on p 135

Example 4 *Calculate the required amount of i cocaine 2% stock solution   ii distilled water to make 70 mL of cocaine solution 1%.*

$$\begin{bmatrix} \text{Amount of} \\ \text{stock} \\ \text{required} \end{bmatrix} = \frac{\text{Strength required}}{\text{Stock strength}} \times \begin{bmatrix} \text{Total volume} \\ \text{required} \end{bmatrix}$$

$$= \frac{1\%}{2\%} \times 70 \text{ mL}$$

$$= \frac{1}{2} \times \frac{70}{1} \text{ mL}$$

$$= 35 \text{ mL}$$

Answer: i 35 mL cocaine 2%   *ii* 35 mL water

Example 5 *A patient is to have a leg bathed in sterile normal saline. Four litre of normal saline solution (0.9%) are to be prepared. What volume of stock 18% saline must be used? What volume of water?*

$$\begin{bmatrix} \text{Amount of} \\ \text{stock} \\ \text{required} \end{bmatrix} = \frac{\text{Strength required}}{\text{Stock strength}} \times \begin{bmatrix} \text{Total volume} \\ \text{required} \end{bmatrix}$$

$$= \frac{0.9\%}{18\%} \times 4 \text{ litre}$$

$$= \frac{0.9}{18} \times \frac{4000}{1} \text{ litre}$$

$$= \frac{9}{180} \times \frac{4000}{1} \text{ mL}$$

$$= 200 \text{ mL}$$

Answer: 200 mL 18% saline, 3800 mL water

Exercise 4B *Calculate the required amounts of stock solution and distilled water to make the following solutions:*

1 0.2 litre of cocaine solution 1% from cocaine 2%

2 35 mL of cocaine solution 1% from cocaine 2%

3 200 mL of cetrimide 1% from concentrated cetrimide 40%

4 Half a litre of cetrimide 1% from concentrated cetrimide 40%

5 500 mL of 1% hypochlorite solution from 10% hypochlorite solution

6 One litre of $2\frac{1}{2}$ % hypochlorite solution from 10% hypochlorite solution

7 **a** One litre **b** 2 litre **c** 1.2 litre of normal saline (0.9%) from 18% saline

8 **a** 500 mL **b** 750 mL **c** $2\frac{1}{2}$ litre of normal saline (0.9%) from 4.5% saline.

Check your answers on p 135

Example 6   *600 mL of lotion, strength 1 in 80, is to be prepared from stock lotion of strength 1 in 20. How much stock lotion is needed? How much water?*

Study this calculation carefully

$$\begin{bmatrix} \text{Amount of} \\ \text{stock} \\ \text{required} \end{bmatrix} = \frac{\text{Strength required}}{\text{Stock strength}} \times \begin{bmatrix} \text{Total volume} \\ \text{required} \end{bmatrix}$$

$$= \frac{1 \text{ in } 80}{1 \text{ in } 20} \times 600 \text{ mL}$$

$$= \frac{1}{80} \div \frac{1}{20} \times \frac{600}{1} \text{ mL}$$

$$= \frac{1}{80} \times \frac{20}{1} \times \frac{600}{1} \text{ mL}$$

$$= 150 \text{ mL}$$

Answer: Stock 150 mL, water 450 mL

Example 7   *$1\frac{1}{2}$ litre of aqueous chlorhexidine 1 : 5000 is required for a douche. Stock solution is 2% chlorhexidine. Calculate the required amount of   i stock   ii distilled water.*

Study this calculation carefully

$$\begin{bmatrix} \text{Amount of} \\ \text{stock} \\ \text{required} \end{bmatrix} = \frac{\text{Strength required}}{\text{Stock strength}} \times \begin{bmatrix} \text{Total volume} \\ \text{required} \end{bmatrix}$$

$$= \frac{1 : 5000}{2\%} \times 1\frac{1}{2} \text{ litre}$$

$$= \frac{1}{5000} \div \frac{2}{100} \times \frac{1500}{1} \text{ mL}$$

$$= \frac{1}{5000} \times \frac{100}{2} \times \frac{1500}{1} \text{ mL}$$

$$= 15 \text{ mL}$$

Answer: Stock 15 mL, water 1485 mL

Note: for practical purposes, write 1 : 5000 as $\frac{1}{5000}$ (rather than $\frac{1}{5001}$)

Exercise 4C *Calculate the amounts of stock solution and distilled water to make the following solutions:*

1 One litre of lotion, strength 1 in 50, from stock lotion of strength 1 in 10

2 $1\frac{1}{2}$ litre of lotion, strength 1 in 150, from stock lotion of strength 1 in 25

3 500 mL of chlorhexidine 1 in 2000 from stock chlorhexidine of strength 1 in 1000

4 1.5 litre of chlorhexidine 1 in 2000 from stock chlorhexidine 1 in 1000

5 600 mL of chlorhexidine 1 in 5000 from stock chlorhexidine 1 in 1000

6 Three litre of 1 : 5000 solution from stock solution 0.1%

7 2.5 litre of 0.05% solution from stock on hand, diluted 1 : 100

8 Two litre of 1 : 10 000 strength solution from stock solution 0.5%

9 700 mL of aqueous chlorhexidine 1 : 2000 from 5% stock solution

10 0.8 litre of 2% solution from stock solution of strength 1 in 25.

Check your answers on p 135

Example 8 *300 mL of Eusol 1 in 20 is to be prepared from pure Eusol. How much pure Eusol is required? How much water must be added?*

$$\left[\begin{array}{c} \text{Amount of} \\ \text{stock} \\ \text{required} \end{array} \right] = \frac{\text{Strength required}}{\text{Stock strength}} \times \left[\begin{array}{c} \text{Total volume} \\ \text{required} \end{array} \right]$$

$$= \frac{1 \text{ in } 20}{1 \text{ in } 1} \times 300 \text{ mL}$$

$$= \frac{1}{20} \times \frac{300}{1} \text{ mL}$$

$$= 15 \text{ mL}$$

Answer: Eusol 15 mL, water 285 mL

Example 9 *What volume of pure Savlon is needed to prepare $1\frac{1}{2}$ litre of a 2% solution?*

$$\left[\begin{array}{c} \text{Amount of} \\ \text{stock} \\ \text{required} \end{array} \right] = \frac{\text{Strength required}}{\text{Stock strength}} \times \left[\begin{array}{c} \text{Total volume} \\ \text{required} \end{array} \right]$$

$$= \frac{2\%}{100\%} \times 1\frac{1}{2} \text{ litre}$$

$$= \frac{2}{100} \times \frac{1500}{1} \text{ mL} \quad \left[\begin{array}{c} \text{percentage signs} \\ \text{cancel out} \end{array} \right]$$

$$= 30 \text{ mL}$$

Answer: Savlon 30 mL

Exercise 4D   *What quantity of **pure** stock is required to make up the following solutions? How much water must be added?*

(Remember that *pure* stock has a strength of *one*. This may be written as just 1 *or* 1 in 1 *or* $\frac{1}{1}$ *or* 100%)

1 800 mL of 5% solution

2 1.5 litre of 10% solution

3 5 L of 1% chlorhexidine solution

4 $2\frac{1}{2}$ litre of 10% chlorhexidine solution

5 One litre of 5% Savlon solution

6 1.2 litre of $2\frac{1}{2}$ % Savlon solution

7 350 mL of 1% Savlon solution

8 1 L of thymol 1 in 8 solution

9 300 mL of thymol 1 : 8 solution

10 100 mL of Eusol solution 1 : 16

Check your answers on p 135

Note: in these examples, percentage strength is generally used to denote grams of solute per 100 mL of water (since 100 mL of water weighs 100 gram).

Example 10   *What weight of sodium bicarbonate is needed to prepare 200 mL of a 5% solution to be used as a mouthwash?*

5% of 200 mL = 5% of 200 gram
[since 200mL water weighs 200 g]

$$= \frac{5}{100} \times \frac{200}{1} \text{ g}$$

$$= 10 \text{ g}$$

Answer: 10 g of sodium bicarbonate

Example 11   *What weight of salbutamol is required to make 2 mL of a 0.5% salbutamol solution?*

0.5% of 2 mL = 0.5% of 2 g
[since 2 mL water weighs 2 g]

$$= \frac{0.5}{100} \times 2000 \text{ mg}$$

$$= \frac{5}{1000} \times \frac{2000}{1} \text{ mg}$$

$$= 10 \text{ mg}$$

Answer: 10 mg of salbutamol

Exercise 4E

1 How many milligrams of chlorpromazine are present in 2 mL of 5% solution?

2 What weight of salbutamol is present in 10 mL of 0.5% solution?

3 How much dextrose is dissolved in
   a 600 mL of 5% solution
   b $1\frac{1}{2}$ litre of 5% solution
   c Half a litre of 2% solution?

4 How many grams of sodium bicarbonate are needed to make
   a 2 litre of a 5% solution
   b 3 litre of $2\frac{1}{2}$ % solution
   c 1 litre of an 8.4% solution?

5 What weight of silver nitrate is dissolved in 300 mL of 5% solution?

6 What volume of *pure* ammonia is required to make
   a 250 mL of 40% ammonia solution
   b 500 mL of 25% ammonia solution?

7 Express as percentage strengths
   a 50 mg of solute per mL of water
   b 15 mg of solute per mL of water
   c 2 g of solute per litre of water.

8 What weight of mannitol is required to make 70 mL of 25% mannitol solution?

9 Calculate the weight of xylocaine needed to make 15 mL of 1% xylocaine solution.

Check your answers on p 135–6

CHAPTER 4 **Revision**

1 Find **a** ratio strength **b** percentage strength when 25 mL of concentrated disinfectant is made up to half a litre with water

2 How much dextrose is dissolved in 800 mL of a dextrose 5% solution?

3 What weight of salbutamol is needed to make 3 mL of a 0.5% salbutamol solution?

Calculate the required amounts of stock solution and distilled water to make the following solutions:

4 3 litre of normal saline (0.9%) from stock 18% saline

5 1200 mL of $2\frac{1}{2}$% hypochlorite solution from 10% hypochlorite solution

6 0.6 litre of lotion, strength 1 in 150, from stock lotion of strength 1 in 10

7 900 mL of aqueous chlorhexidine 1 : 2000 from 5% stock solution

8 1.4 L of $2\frac{1}{2}$% Savlon solution from *pure* Savlon

9 600 mL of thymol 1 in 8 solution from *pure* thymol

Check your answers on p 136

5. Intravenous infusion

This chapter deals with the arithmetic of flow rates and drip rates for intravenous (I.V.) infusion.

The fluid being infused passes from a flask (or similar container) into a *drip chamber* or into a *volumetric infusion pump*.

A drip chamber is part of a *giving set* or *administration set*. It has a *fixed* drop size and an *adjustable* rate of flow. There are four main types of giving set in general use – these break fluid into either 10, 15, 20 or 60 drops per mL. A drip chamber which delivers 60 drops per mL is also known as a *microdrip*.

A volumetric infusion pump receives fluid from a giving set. The pump has an *adjustable* rate of flow and converts fluid into very fine drops, within the machine, before delivering the fluid to a patient.

An infusion pump can be accurately set and is designed to maintain a steady flow rate. However, the patient receiving the infusion must still be checked at regular intervals.

Example 1 *A patient is receiving dextrose 5% by I.V. infusion. The drip chamber is set to deliver at a rate of 45 mL per hour. How much fluid will the patient receive over   i 2 h   ii 3 h   iii 7 h?*

Volume (mL)   =   Rate (mL/h) × Time (h)

i   45mL/h × 2 h   =   90 mL
ii   45 mL/h × 3 h   =   135 mL
iii 45 mL/h × 7 h   =   315 mL

Example 2 *A teenager is to receive 750 mL of Hartmann's solution. An infusion pump is set at 60 mL/h. How long will it take to give the solution?*

$$\text{Time (h)} = \frac{\text{Volume (mL)}}{\text{Rate (mL/h)}}$$

$$= \frac{750 \text{ mL}}{60 \text{ mL/h}}$$

$$= 12\tfrac{1}{2} \text{ hours or 12 h 30 min}$$

Exercise 5A

1 An intravenous line has been inserted in a patient. Fluid is being delivered at a steady rate of 40 mL/h. How much fluid will the patient receive in **a** 2 h **b** 8 h **c** 12 h?

2 A male patient is receiving Hartmann's solution from a drip chamber at a rate of 35 mL/h. How much solution will he receive over **a** 3 h **b** 5 h **c** 12 h?

3 A girl is to be given dextrose 5% I.V. If the infusion pump is set at 60 mL/h, how much dextrose 5% will she receive in **a** $1\frac{1}{2}$ h

   b $2\frac{1}{2}$ h **c** 12 h?

4 A female patient is to receive 500 mL of normal saline. The drip chamber is adjusted to deliver 25 mL/h. How long will the fluid last?

5 A young man is to be given one litre of dextrose 4% in $\frac{1}{5}$ normal saline. The infusion pump is set at a rate of 80 mL/h. What time will it take to give the litre of solution?

6 Half a litre of glycine 1.5% is to be given to a patient I.V. How long will this take if the infusion pump is set at 75 mL/h?

7 A patient is to receive 100 mL of normal saline, I.V. If the infusion pump is set to deliver 150 mL/h, how long will the infusion take?

Check your answers on p 136

Example 3 *A patient is to receive half a litre of fluid I.V. over 6 hours using an infusion pump. At what flow rate (in mL/h) should the pump be set? If your answer is a mixed number then go to the next whole number.*

Half a litre $=$ 500 mL

Rate (mL/h) $= \dfrac{\text{Volume (mL)}}{\text{Time (h)}}$

$= \dfrac{500 \text{ mL}}{6 \text{ h}}$

$= 83\frac{1}{3}$ mL/h

$\Rightarrow$ 84 mL/h (using *next whole number*)

Example 4 *500 mL of fluid is dripping at 20 drops/min. The I.V. set delivers 15 drops/mL. How long will it take for the patient to receive the fluid?*

Time (hours) $= \dfrac{\text{Volume (drops)}}{\text{Rate (drops/hour)}}$

$= \dfrac{\text{Volume (drops)}}{\text{Rate (drops/min)} \times 60}$

$= \dfrac{500 \text{ mL} \times 15 \text{ drops/mL}}{20 \text{ drops/min} \times 60}$

$= \dfrac{500 \times 15}{20 \times 60} \text{ h}$

$= 6\frac{1}{4}$ hours or 6 h 15 min

Exercise 5B   *Calculate the required flow rate of a volumetric infusion pump for each of the following infusions. Give answers in mL/h.* **If a calculated answer is a mixed number then go to the next whole number.**

1 One litre of normal saline is to be given over 8 hours

2 A patient is to receive 1500 mL of dextrose 5% over 12 hours

3 500 mL of Hartmann's solution is to be given to a teenager over 7 hours

4 Over the next 15 hours, a female patient is to receive two litre of dextrose 4% in $\frac{1}{5}$ normal saline

5 A young man is to be given $1\frac{1}{2}$ L of glycine 1.5% over 8 hours.

Exercise 5C   *Calculate how long each infusion will take:*

1 One litre of fluid is to drip at 50 drops per minute. The I.V. set delivers 15 drops per mL

2 750 mL of normal saline is being given at 25 drops/min, 20 drops/mL

3 A microdrip delivers 60 drops/mL. A young patient is to receive 250 mL of dextrose 5% at 30 drops/min

4 A patient is to have one litre of Hartmann's solution. The giving set delivers 10 drops/mL at a rate of 25 drops/min

5 A litre of glycine 1.5% is to be given I.V. The administration set gives 15 drops/mL and is adjusted to 40 drops/min.

Check your answers on p 137

Example 5 *800 mL of fluid is to be given over 5 hours. The I.V. set delivers 15 drops per mL. At what rate (in drops per minute) should it drip?*

$$\text{Rate (drops/min)} = \frac{\text{Volume (drops)}}{\text{Time (minutes)}}$$

$$= \frac{\text{Volume (drops)}}{\text{Time (hours)} \times 60}$$

$$= \frac{800 \text{ mL} \times 15 \text{ drops/mL}}{5 \text{ h} \times 60}$$

$$= \frac{800 \times 15}{5 \times 60} \text{ drops/min}$$

$$= 40 \text{ drops/min}$$

Example 6 *A patient is to receive half a litre of dextrose 5% over 4 hours. The giving set delivers 20 drops/mL. Calculate the required drip rate in drops/min. If the answer is a mixed number then go to the next whole number.*

$$\text{Half a litre} = 500 \text{ mL}$$

$$\text{Rate (drops/min)} = \frac{\text{Volume (drops)}}{\text{Time (minutes)}}$$

$$= \frac{\text{Volume (drops)}}{\text{Time (hours)} \times 60}$$

$$= \frac{500 \text{ mL} \times 20 \text{ drops/mL}}{4 \text{ h} \times 60}$$

$$= \frac{500 \times 20}{4 \times 60} \text{ drops/min}$$

$$= \frac{125}{3} \text{ drops/min}$$

$$= 41\tfrac{2}{3} \text{ drops/min}$$

$$\Rightarrow 42 \text{ drops/min}$$
(using *next whole number*)

Example 7   *At 0600 hours, a one litre flask of normal saline is set up to run through an infusion pump at 70 mL/h. After 8 hours, the flow rate is increased to 80 mL/h. By what time would the flask have to be replaced?*

i   Volume (mL)   = Rate (mL/h) × Time (h)

    = 70 mL/h × 8 h

    = 560 mL

ii   One litre   = 1000 mL

    ∴ Volume remaining = 1000 mL − 560 mL

    = 440 mL

iii   Time (hours)   = $\dfrac{\text{Volume (mL)}}{\text{Rate (mL/h)}}$

    = $\dfrac{440 \text{ mL}}{80 \text{ mL/h}}$

    = $5\frac{1}{2}$ h or 5 h 30 min

iv   Total running time   = 8 h + $5\frac{1}{2}$ h

    = $13\frac{1}{2}$ h or 13 h 30 min

    ∴ Finishing time   = 0600 h + 13 h 30 min

    = 1930 h

Exercise 5D *Calculate the required drip rate in drops per minute. If the answer to a drip rate calculation is a mixed number, then use the next whole number for practical purposes, and to ensure that the infusion is completed in the given time.*

1 An infant is ordered 150 mL of Hartmann's solution to run over 6 hours. The microdrip delivers 60 drops per mL.

2 A teenager is to receive 500 mL of dextrose 5% over 8 hours. The I.V. set emits 20 drops/mL.

3 0.5 litre of dextrose 4% in $\frac{1}{5}$ normal saline is to run over 12 hours. The administration set delivers 15 drops/mL.

4 750 mL of normal saline is to be given to a patient over 9 hours using a giving set which emits 10 drops/mL.

5 An adult male is to be given half a litre of glycine 1.5% over 5 hours using an I.V. set which gives 15 drops per mL.

6 A female patient is to receive $1\frac{1}{2}$ litre of fluid over 10 hours. The giving set delivers 20 drops/mL.

7 A patient in intensive care is to have the remaining 300 mL of dextrose 5% run through in 50 minutes. The administration set gives 15 drops/mL.

Check your answers on p 137

Exercise 5E   *Blood and blood products are infused using a drip chamber which delivers either 10 drops/mL or 15 drops/mL. A microdrip must **not** be used to infuse either blood or blood products. Calculate the drip rate in drops/min. Assume that one unit contains 500 mL. If an answer is a mixed number then go to the **next whole number**.*

1 An anaemic child must be given one unit of packed cells over 5 hours. The I.V. set delivers 15 drops/mL.

2 An anaemic adult male is to be given 2 units of blood in 8 hours. The giving set emits 15 drops/mL.

3 Towards the end of a transfusion, a woman has still to be given $1\frac{1}{2}$ units of blood over 5 hours. The I.V. set delivers 15 drops/mL.

4 300 mL of blood is to be transfused over 4 hours using an administration set which gives 10 drops/mL.

5 One unit of packed red cells is to be run over 3 hours. An I.V. set which emits 10 drops/mL is to be used.

6 A patient is to be given one unit of plasma over 6 hours using a giving set which delivers 15 drops/mL.

Check your answers on p 137

Exercise 5F

1 A patient has *two* intravenous lines inserted. One line is running at 45 mL/h; the other at 30 mL/h. What volume of fluid would this patient receive in a 24-hour period?

2 One litre of Hartmann's solution is to be given I.V. For the first 6 hours the solution is delivered at 85 mL/h, then the rate is reduced to 70 mL/h. Find the total time taken to give the full volume.

3 A patient is to receive half a litre of dextrose 5% I.V. A flask is set up at 0800 hours running at 60 mL/h. After 5 hours the rate is increased to 80 mL/h. At what time will the I.V. be completed?

4 At 0430 hours, an infusion pump is set to deliver 1.5 litres of fluid at a rate of 90 mL/h. After 10 hours the pump is reset to 75 mL/h. Calculate the finishing time.

5 A 1 litre I.V. flask of normal saline has been running for 6 hours at a rate of 75 mL/h. The doctor orders the remaining contents to be run through in the next 5 hours. Calculate the new flow rate.

6 A patient is to receive one litre of dextrose 4% in $\frac{1}{5}$ normal saline.

For the first $3\frac{1}{2}$ hours the fluid is delivered at 160 mL/h.

A specialist then orders the rate slowed so that the remaining fluid will be run over the next 8 hours. Calculate the required flow rate.

Check your answers on p 137–8

Example 8   *One gram of dextrose provides 16 kilojoules of energy. How many kilojoules does a patient receive from an infusion of $1\frac{1}{2}$ litres of 10% dextrose?*

10% dextrose = 10 g of dextrose per 100 mL of solution

$$= \frac{10 \text{ g}}{100 \text{ mL}}$$

$1\frac{1}{2}$ litres = 1500 mL

Weight of dextrose = Volume of infusion × strength of solution

$$= \frac{1500 \text{ mL} \times 10 \text{ g}}{100 \text{ mL}}$$

= 15 × 10 g   [1500 mL ÷ 100 mL = 15]

= 150 g

Energy supplied = 150 g × 16 kJ/g

= 2400 kJ

The symbol for kilojoules is kJ

Exercise 5G   *One gram of carbohydrate provides 16 kilojoules of energy. Dextrose and glucose are carbohydrates. Calculate how many kilojoules are supplied to a patient in each of the following infusions.*

1 One litre of 5% dextrose

2 $2\frac{1}{2}$ L of 5% dextrose

3 One litre of 10% dextrose

4 500 mL of 20% dextrose

5 Two litre of normal saline

Normal saline is a 0.9% solution of salt in water.

6 750 mL of 4% dextrose in $\frac{1}{5}$ normal saline

7 $1\frac{1}{2}$ L of Hartmann's solution.

Hartmann's solution contains sodium lactate, sodium chloride, potassium chloride, and calcium chloride.

8 A diabetic patient is found unconscious and presumed to be hypoglycaemic. 50 mL of 50% glucose is given to the patient. How many kilojoules of energy are administered in the 50 mL dose?

Check your answers on p 138

CHAPTER 5   **Revision**

1 A male patient is receiving dextrose 5% from a drip chamber at a rate of 55 mL/h. How much fluid will he receive in
   a 2 h   **b** 5 h   **c** 11 h?

2 A patient is to receive one litre of Hartmann's solution. If an infusion pump is set at 120 mL/h, how long will the pump take to give the solution?

3 1.5 litre of dextrose 4% in $\frac{1}{5}$ normal saline is to be given to a patient over 20 hours. Calculate the required flow rate setting for a volumetric infusion pump.

4 An infusion pump is to be used to give 1 L of fluid over 11 hours. At what flow rate should the pump be set?

5 750 mL of fluid is being given at 30 drops per minute. The drip chamber delivers 15 drops per mL. How long will the fluid last at this drip rate?

6 A patient is to be given $1\frac{1}{2}$ litre of fluid over 10 hours. The giving set emits 20 drops/mL. Calculate the required drip rate in drops/min.

7 A female patient is to receive one litre of Hartmann's solution over 12 hours. Calculate the drip rate if the administration set gives 15 drops/mL.

8 A patient is receiving fluid from *two* I.V. lines. One line is running at 65 mL/h; the other at 70 mL/h. What volume of fluid would the patient receive I.V. over 12 hours?

9 A litre of dextrose 5% is to be given I.V. The solution is to run at 75 mL/h for the first 6 hours, then the rate reduced to 50 mL/h. Calculate the total time required to give the full volume.

Check your answers on p 138

10 At 0300 hours, two litre of normal saline is set running through an infusion pump at 85 mL/h. After 8 hours the rate is increased to 120 mL/h. Calculate the finishing time.

11 A one litre I.V. flask of glycine 1.5% has been running at 90 mL/h for 6 hours. A specialist then orders the rate speeded up so that the remaining solution will be run through in the next 4 hours. Calculate the new flow rate in mL/h.

12 One gram of dextrose provides 16 kJ of energy. How many kilojoules does a patient receive from an infusion of $1\frac{1}{2}$ L of 5% dextrose?

Check your answers on p 138

6. Paediatric dosages (body weight)

Most drug dosages are based on the weight of a patient (although, for some groups of drugs, the dosages are based on body surface area — see Chapter 7).

Figure 6.1 shows the age and average weight of males and females.

Great care must be taken when dispensing drugs for children as their range of weights is so wide. When dosages are prescribed in *micrograms*, write that unit *in full*, to avoid confusion and prevent overdoses.

Overdoses can be fatal.

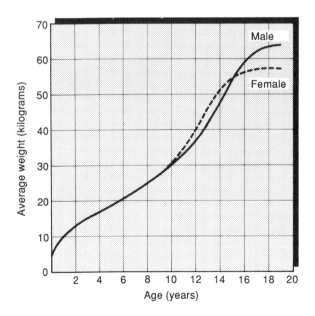

Fig. 6.1   Age and average weight of males and females.

Example 1 *A child is prescribed erythromycin. The recommended dosage is 40 mg/kg/day, 4 doses daily. If the child's weight is 15 kg, calculate the size of a single dose.*

$$
\begin{array}{rl}
15 & \text{kg} \\
\times\ 40 & \text{mg/kg/day} \\
\hline
4\overline{)600} & \text{mg/day} \\
\hline
150 & \text{mg/dose} \\
\hline
\end{array}
$$

Example 2 *A child is to be given ampicillin. The recommended dosage is 80 mg/kg/day, 4 doses per day. Calculate the size of a single dose if the child's weight is 27 kg.*

$$
\begin{array}{rl}
27 & \text{kg} \\
\times\quad 80 & \text{mg/kg/day} \\
\hline
4\overline{)2160} & \text{mg/day} \\
\hline
540 & \text{mg/dose} \\
\hline
\end{array}
$$

Exercise 6A   *Calculate single doses according to each child's body weight.*

Calculate the size of a single dose for a child weighing 12 kg:
1 Erythromycin, 40 mg/kg/day, 4 doses per day
2 Penicillin V, 50 mg/kg/day, 4 doses per day
3 Cephalexin, 30 mg/kg/day, 4 doses per day

Calculate the size of a single dose for a child weighing 20 kg:
4 Cloxacillin, 50 mg/kg/day, 4 doses per day
5 Chloramphenicol, 40 mg/kg/day, 4 doses per day
6 Amoxicillin, 45 mg/kg/day, 4 doses per day

Calculate the size of a single dose for a child weighing 36 kg:
7 Methicillin, 100 mg/kg/day, 4 doses per day
8 Capreomycin sulphate, 20 mg/kg/day, 3 doses per day
9 Cephalothin, 60 mg/kg/day, 4 doses per day

Check your answers on p 138

Example 3   *A boy is ordered pethidine 35 mg, I.M. Stock ampoules contain 50 mg in 1 mL. What volume must be withdrawn for injection?*

$$\begin{aligned}\text{Volume}\atop\text{required}\end{aligned} = \frac{\text{Strength required}}{\text{Stock strength}} \times \left[\begin{aligned}\text{Volume of}\\\text{stock solution}\end{aligned}\right]$$

$$= \frac{35 \text{ mg}}{50 \text{ mg}} \times 1 \text{ mL}$$

$$= \frac{7}{10} \text{ mL or } 0.7 \text{ mL}$$

Example 4   *An infant needs a maintenance injection of digoxin 40 microgram. Paediatric ampoules contain 50 µg/2 mL. Calculate the amount to be drawn up.*

$$\begin{aligned}\text{Volume}\atop\text{required}\end{aligned} = \frac{\text{Strength required}}{\text{Stock strength}} \times \left[\begin{aligned}\text{Volume of}\\\text{stock solution}\end{aligned}\right]$$

$$= \frac{40 \text{ microgram}}{50 \text{ microgram}} \times 2 \text{ mL}$$

$$= \frac{8}{5} \text{ mL or } 1.6 \text{ mL}$$

Example 5   *A child with TB is to be given 125 mg of capreomycin sulphate by I.M.I. Stock on hand has a strength of 1 g in 2 mL. What volume of stock must be injected?*

$$\begin{aligned}\text{Volume}\atop\text{required}\end{aligned} = \frac{\text{Strength required}}{\text{Stock strength}} \times \left[\begin{aligned}\text{Volume of}\\\text{stock solution}\end{aligned}\right]$$

$$= \frac{125 \text{ mg}}{1000 \text{ mg}} \times 2 \text{ mL}$$

$$= \frac{25}{100} \text{ mL or } 0.25 \text{ mL}$$

Exercise 6B   *Calculate the volume to be withdrawn for injection for each of these paediatric dosages.*

	Ordered		Stock ampoule
1	Pethidine	20 mg	50 mg in 1 mL
2	Cortisone	10 mg	25 mg in 1 mL
3	Cortisone	20 mg	50 mg in 2 mL
4	Atropine	0.3 mg	0.4 mg in 1 mL
5	Digoxin	125 microgram	0.5 mg/2 mL
6	Digoxin	18 microgram	50 µg in 2 mL
7	Capreomycin sulphate	200 mg	1 gram in 2 mL
8	Capreomycin sulphate	150 mg	1 gram in 5 mL
9	Kanamycin	120 mg	500 mg in 2 mL
10	Kanamycin	300 mg	500 mg in 2 mL
11	Methicillin	400 mg	1 g in 3 mL
12	Sulphadimidine	100 mg	1 g in 3 mL
13	Phenobarbitone	50 mg	200 mg/mL
14	Phenobarbitone	120 mg	200 mg/mL
15	Morphine	6.5 mg	10 mg in 1 mL
16	Gentamicin	15 mg	20 mg/2 mL
17	Gentamicin	40 mg	60 mg/1.5 mL
18	Chlorpromazine	8 mg	10 mg/mL
19	Chlorpromazine	15 mg	25 mg/mL
20	Omnopon	16 mg	20 mg per mL

Check your answers on p 139

Example 6 *A child is ordered 80 mg of paracetamol elixir. Stock on hand is 100 mg in 5 mL. Calculate the volume to be given.*

$$\text{Volume required} = \frac{\text{Strength required}}{\text{Stock strength}} \times \left[\begin{array}{c} \text{Volume of} \\ \text{stock solution} \end{array} \right]$$

$$= \frac{80 \text{ mg}}{100 \text{ mg}} \times 5 \text{ mL}$$

$$= 4 \text{ mL}$$

Example 7 *A child is to be given 175 microgram of digoxin, orally. Paediatric mixture contains 50 microgram per mL. Calculate the required volume.*

$$\text{Volume required} = \frac{\text{Strength required}}{\text{Stock strength}} \times \left[\begin{array}{c} \text{Volume of} \\ \text{stock solution} \end{array} \right]$$

$$= \frac{175 \text{ microgram}}{50 \text{ microgram}} \times 1 \text{ mL}$$

$$= \frac{7}{2} \text{ mL or 3.5 mL}$$

Example 8 *A child is prescribed 180 mg of aspirin. On hand is a mixture containing 150 mg in 5 mL. How much should be given?*

$$\text{Volume required} = \frac{\text{Strength required}}{\text{Stock strength}} \times \left[\begin{array}{c} \text{Volume of} \\ \text{stock solution} \end{array} \right]$$

$$= \frac{180 \text{ mg}}{150 \text{ mg}} \times 5 \text{ mL}$$

$$= 6 \text{ mL}$$

Exercise 6C   *Calculate the volume to be given orally for these paediatric dosages. (The strength of the stock mixture is given in brackets)*

1 70 mg of paracetamol elixir
(100 mg/5 mL)

2 300 mg of paracetamol elixir
(120 mg/5 mL)

3 600 mg of sulphadiazine
(500 mg/5 mL)

4 900 mg of sulphadiazine
(500 mg/5 mL)

5 125 microgram of digoxin
(50 microgram/mL)

6 200 mg of penicillin
(125 mg/5 mL)

7 350 mg of penicillin
(125 mg/5 mL)

8 15 mg of chlorpromazine
(25 mg/5 mL)

9 120 mg of aspirin
(150 mg/5 mL)

10 200 mg of aspirin
(150 mg/5 mL)

11 50 mg of amoxycillin
(1 g/10 mL)

12 100 mg of flucloxacillin
(125 mg/5 mL)

Check your answers on p 139

CHAPTER 6 **Revision**

1 A child is prescribed cloxacillin. The recommended dosage is 50 mg/kg/day; 4 doses daily. Calculate the size of a *single* dose if the child's weight is 22 kg.

2 A young boy weighing 19 kg is to be given cephalothin. The recommended dosage is 60 mg/kg/day; 4 doses daily. What should be the size of a *single* dose?

3 The recommended dosage for capreomycin sulphate is 20 mg/kg/day; 3 doses daily. Calculate the size of a *single* dose for a girl weighing 27 kg.

4 A girl is ordered cortisone 15 mg. Stock ampoules on hand contain 50 mg in 2 mL. What volume must be withdrawn for injection?

5 A child is prescribed methicillin 320 mg. Ampoules contain methicillin 1 gram in 3 mL. What volume should be injected?

6 An infant requires an injection of digoxin 45 microgram. Calculate the amount to be drawn up if paediatric ampoules contain 50 microgram/2 mL.

7 A child is to be given 180 mg of paracetamol. Stock elixir contains 120 mg/5 mL. Calculate the volume to be given orally.

8 A boy is prescribed 800 mg sulphadiazine, to be taken orally. What volume of mixture should be given if stock mixture contains 500 mg in 5 mL?

9 A young patient is ordered penicillin 300 mg. Mixture on hand has a strength of 125 mg/5 mL. How much mixture should be given?

Check your answers on p 139

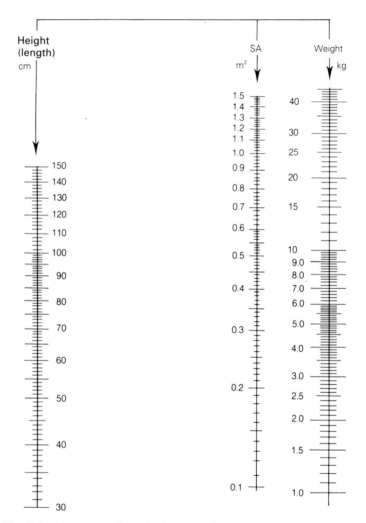

Fig. 7.1 Nomogram for calculating surface area. Surface area (S.A.) is shown when height (or length) and weight are linked by a straight line (use a ruler).

7. Paediatric dosages (surface area)

As mentioned previously, the dosages for some groups of drugs are based on *body surface area*. The drugs involved are used in critical care situations. Body surface area has a major effect on heat loss and moisture loss from the body.

The nomogram (Fig. 7.1 on the opposite page) is a graph which relates a person's height (or length), weight and surface area. Once the height and weight of a patient have been measured then the body surface area can be determined using the nomogram.

Children of the same age have a wide range of heights and weights and, consequently, a wide range of surface areas.

Example 1 *Using the nomogram at the beginning of this chapter, find the body surface area of a 6-month-old infant with a length of 65 cm and weight of 8.2 kg.*

On the nomogram, join length 65 cm and weight 8.2 kg with a straight edge (e.g. ruler). The straight edge then crosses the surface area scale (marked S.A.) at 0.40 m^2.

Example 2 *Using the nomogram, determine the body surface area of a 2-year-old boy of length 87 cm and weight 13.5 kg.*

On the nomogram, join length 87 cm and weight 13.5 kg with a straight edge. The straight edge then crosses the surface area scale at 0.58 m^2.

Exercise 7A   *The lengths and weights used below represent children from 3 months to 3 years of age. Use the nomogram to find the body surface area of each child. Estimate answers to the nearest 0.01 m².*

1 **a** Length 65 cm, weight 6.4 kg
   b Length 65 cm, weight 8.2 kg

2 **a** Length 73 cm, weight 8.8 kg
   b Length 73 cm, weight 10.5 kg

3 **a** Length 85 cm, weight 11.0 kg
   b Length 85 cm, weight 13.5 kg

4 **a** Length 94 cm, weight 12.5 kg
   b Length 94 cm, weight 15.5 kg

5 **a** Weight 5.7 kg, length 57 cm
   b Weight 5.7 kg, length 63 cm

6 **a** Weight 9.4 kg, length 68 cm
   b Weight 9.4 kg, length 74 cm

7 **a** Weight 11.5 kg, length 78 cm
   b Weight 11.5 kg, length 86 cm

8 **a** Weight 14.0 kg, length 87 cm
   b Weight 14.0 kg, length 97 cm

Check your answers on p 139

Example 3 *A young leukaemia patient is to be given his weekly injection of doxorubicin. The recommended dosage is 30 mg/m² and the boy's body surface area has been determined at 0.48 m². Stock solution contains doxorubicin 10 mg/5 mL. Calculate volume to be drawn up for injection.*

0.48	m²	Body surface area
× 30	mg/m²	Recommended dosage
14.40	mg	Dose required

$$\text{Volume required} = \frac{\text{Dose required}}{\text{Stock strength}} \times \left[\begin{array}{c} \text{Volume of} \\ \text{stock solution} \end{array} \right]$$

$$= \frac{14.4 \text{ mg}}{10 \text{ mg}} \times 5 \text{ mL}$$

$$= 7.2 \text{ mL}$$

Exercise 7B   *The aim of this exercise is to introduce the method of calculating drug doses based on body surface areas. These doses are used in critical care situations, such as the treatment of children with leukaemia, and are administered under very strict procedures and supervision. Calculate the volume required in each case.*

1 *Prescribed*: dactinomycin
   Recommended dosage: 1.5 mg/m^2
   Stock strength: 500 microgram/mL
   Body surface area: 0.40 m^2

2 *Prescribed*: bleomycin
   Recommended dosage: 10 units/m^2
   Stock strength: 15 U/5 mL
   Body surface area: 0.54 m^2

3 *Prescribed*: cytarabine
   Recommended dosage: 120 mg/m^2
   Stock strength: 100 mg/5 mL
   Body surface area: 0.45 m^2

4 *Prescribed*: daunorubicin
   Recommended dosage: 30 mg/m^2
   Stock strength: 20 mg/5 mL
   Body surface area: 0.52 m^2

5 *Prescribed*: vincristine
   Recommended dosage: 1.5 mg/m^2
   Stock strength: 1 mg/mL
   Body surface area: 0.64 m^2

Check your answers on p 139

CHAPTER 7 **Revision**

Use the nomogram to work out the answers to questions 1–4:

1 Find the body surface area of a 4-year-old girl of height 102 cm and weight 16.5 kg.

2 A 5-year-old boy has a height of 108 cm and he weighs 18.5 kg. Find his surface area.

3 A girl is 7 years old. Her height is 120 cm and weight 20.5 kg. What is her surface area?

4 An 8-year-old boy weighs 24 kg and has a height of 124 cm. Determine his surface area.

5 A boy is to be given bleomycin I.M.I. The recommended dosage is 10 units per m^2. Reconstituted stock has a strength of 15 U/5 mL. What volume should be injected if the boy has a surface area of 0.48 m^2?

6 A young patient is prescribed doxorubicin. The recommended dosage is 30 mg/m^2 and stock contains 50 mg/25 mL. Calculate the volume required if the patient's surface area is 0.70 m^2.

Check your answers on p 140

8. Summary exercises

Summary exercise I

1 A patient is prescribed methicillin 1200 mg, I.M.I. Stock ampoules contain 1 gram in 5 mL. Is the volume to be drawn up for injection equal to 5 mL, less than 5 mL, or more than 5 mL?

2 A patient is ordered erythromycin 135 mg, I.M.I. Stock vials contain 300 mg/10 mL. Calculate the volume required for injection.

3 300 000 units of benzathine penicillin are to be given by I.M.I. On hand is benzathine penicillin 1.2 megaunits in 2 mL. What volume should be drawn up?

4 450 mg of soluble aspirin is required. Stock on hand is 300 mg tablets. How many tablets should be given?

5 Warfarin tablets are available in strengths of 1 mg, 2 mg, 5 mg and 10 mg. Choose the best combination of whole tablets for each of the following dosages of warfarin **a** 4 mg **b** 8 mg **c** 12 mg.

6 A patient is ordered 360 mg of penicillin, orally. The strength of the stock syrup is 125 mg/5 mL. Calculate the volume required.

7 A solution has a strength of $12\frac{1}{2}$ %. Express $12\frac{1}{2}$ % as a *ratio* strength.

8 5 litre of normal saline solution (0.9%) is to be prepared. What volume of **a** stock 18% saline **b** water must be used?

9 Calculate the amount of **a** stock solution **b** distilled water, to make $12\frac{1}{2}$ litre of lotion, strength 1 in 50, from stock lotion of strength 1 in 10.

Check your answers on p 140

10 1.2 litre of thymol 1 in 8 is to be prepared.
   a What quantity of *pure* stock is required?
   b How much water must be added?

11 How many grams of sodium bicarbonate should be used to prepared 2 litre of a $2\frac{1}{2}$ % solution?

12 A male patient is receiving dextrose 5% from a giving set at a rate of 25 mL/h. How much of the solution will he receive over
   a 3 h   **b** 5 h   **c** 12 h?

13 One litre of Hartmann's solution is to be given over 12 hours. Calculate the required flow rate of a volumetric infusion pump.

14 700 mL of Hartmann's solution is to be given over 8 hours. The I.V. set delivers 15 drops/mL. At what rate should it drip?

15 800 mL of fluid is to be given I.V. The fluid is run at 70 mL/h for the first 5 hours then the rate is reduced to 60 mL/h. Find the total time taken to give the 800 mL.

16 One gram of dextrose provides 16 kJ of energy. How many kilojoules does a patient receive from an infusion of half a litre of 10% dextrose?

17 A child is prescribed penicillin V. The recommended dosage is 50 mg/kg/day; 4 doses daily. If the child's weight is 18 kg, calculate the size of a single dose.

18 A girl is ordered phenobarbitone 140 mg. Stock ampoules contain 200 mg/mL. What volume must be withdrawn for injection?

19 A child is prescribed 175 mg capreomycin sulphate by I.M.I. A stock ampoule contains 1 g in 2 mL. What volume of stock must be injected?

20 A young boy is to have 125 microgram of digoxin, orally. Paediatric mixture has a strength of 50 microgram per mL. Calculate the required volume.

Check your answers on p 140

21 Using the nomogram, find the body surface area of a 9-month-old-girl of length 68 cm and weight 9.2 kg.

22 A child is prescribed dactinomycin I.V. The recommended dosage is 0.9 mg/m^2 and stock on hand has a strength of 500 microgram/mL. Calculate the volume to be injected if the child's surface area is 0.55 m^2.

Check your answers on p 140

Summary exercise II

1 Capreomycin sulphate 900 mg is ordered. Stock ampoules contain 1 gram in 3 mL. Is the volume required for injection equal to 3 mL, less than 3 mL, or more than 3 mL?

2 An injection of digoxin 225 microgram is ordered. Stock on hand is digoxin 500 microgram in 2 mL. What volume of stock should be given?

3 How many 30 mg tablets of phenobarbitone should be given if phenobarbitone 15 mg is prescribed?

4 Thioridazine tablets are available in strengths of 10 mg, 25 mg, 50 mg and 100 mg. What combination of tablets should be used for the following dosages **a** 60 mg **b** 85 mg **c** 110 mg?

5 900 mg of benzyl penicillin is to be given orally. Stock mixture contains 250 mg/5 mL. Calculate the volume of mixture to be given.

6 Calculate the percentage strength when 5 mL of disinfectant concentrate is mixed with water to make 1 litre of solution.

7 Calculate the percentage strength of the solution made by dissolving 20 g of dextrose in 500 mL of water.

8 600 mL of cetrimide 1% is required. What volume of **a** concentrated cetrimide 40% **b** distilled water should be used?

9 Calculate the amount of **a** stock solution **b** distilled water to make 800 mL of chlorhexidine 1 : 2000 from 2% stock solution.

10 What volume of pure Savlon is needed to prepare 2.4 litre of a 5% solution? How much water must be added?

11 What weight of dextrose is required to make 1500 mL of dextrose 5% solution?

12 A patient is to receive one litre of normal saline, I.V.I. The infusion pump is set at 80 mL/h. How long will the fluid last?

Check your answers on p 141

13 Over the next 9 hours, a patient is to be given half a litre of dextrose 4% in $\frac{1}{5}$ normal saline using a volumetric infusion pump. At what flow rate should the pump be set?

14 750 mL of dextrose 5% is dripping at 30 drops/min. The I.V. set delivers 15 drops/mL. How long will it take for the patient to receive this fluid?

15 A patient is to be given 1.2 litre of fluid, I.V.I. An infusion pump is set at a rate of 60 mL/h. After 12 hours the rate is increased to 96 mL/h. Calculate the total running time.

16 One gram of dextrose provides 16 kJ of energy. A patient is given an infusion of two litre of 4% dextrose in $\frac{1}{5}$ normal saline. How many kilojoules does this infusion provide?

17 A child is to be given capreomycin sulphate. The recommended dosage is 20 mg/kg/day; 3 doses per day. Calculate the size of a single dose if the child's weight is 24 kg.

18 It is necessary to give an infant an injection of digoxin 35 microgram. Paediatric ampoules contain 50 µg/2 mL. Calculate the amount to be drawn up.

19 A boy is ordered 120 mg of paracetamol elixir. Stock on hand has a strength of 100 mg/5 mL. What volume should be given?

20 A young girl is prescribed 700 mg of sulphadiazine, to be taken orally. The stock mixture contains 500 mg/5 mL. How much mixture should be given?

21 Using the nomogram, determine the body surface area of a 2-year-old boy whose length is 87 cm and weight 13.5 kg.

22 A young girl is to be given cytarabine I.V. The recommended dosage is 150 mg/m^2. The girl's surface area is found to be 0.60 m^2. Stock on hand has a strength of 500 mg/5 mL. What volume should be drawn up for injection?

Check your answers on p 141

ANSWERS TO DIAGNOSTIC TEST

		Reference Exercise
1	a 830 b 8300 c 83 000	1A
2	a 0.258 b 2.58 c 25.8	1A
3	a 0.378 b 0.0378 c 0.003 78	1B
4	a 56.9 b 5.69 c 0.569	1B
5	a 1000 b 1000 c 1000	1C
6	a 780 mg b 0.034 g	1C
7	a 86 micrograms b 0.294 mg	1C
8	a 2400 mL b 0.965 L	1C
9	a 70 mL b 7 mL c 0.07 L is larger	1D
10	a 45 mg b 450 mg c 0.45 g is heavier	1D
11	a 27 b 2.7 c 0.27 d 0.0027	1E
12	a 468 b 4.68 c 4.68 d 0.468	1E
13	675 mL	1F
14	2150 mL or 2.15 L	1F
15	2, 3, 6, 7 and 9 are factors	1G
16	a $\frac{2}{3}$ b $\frac{7}{9}$	1H
17	a $\frac{3}{40}$ b $\frac{7}{16}$	1H
18	a $\frac{4}{5}$ b $\frac{2}{3}$ c $\frac{3}{5}$	1I
19	a $\frac{7}{10}$ b $\frac{4}{5}$ c $\frac{2}{5}$	1I
20	a 0.7 b 1.8 c 0.4	1J
21	a 0.37 b 2.63 c 0.52	1J
22	a 1.608 b 0.570 c 2.657	1J
23	a 0.625 b 0.45 c 0.68 d 0.775	1K
24	a 0.2 b 0.4 c 0.8	1L
25	a 0.71 b 0.56	1L
26	a 0.233 b 0.843	1L
27	a 75% b 65% c 32%	1M
28	a $33\frac{1}{3}$% b $62\frac{1}{2}$% c $55\frac{5}{9}$%	1M

		Reference *Exercise*
29	**a** 1 in 5 **b** 1 in 21	*1N*
30	**a** 1 : 3 **b** 1 : 29	*1N*
31	200 mL	*1N*
32	80 mL	*1N*
33	**a** 20% **b** 2% **c** 0.2% **d** 0.02%	*1O*
34	**a** $\frac{3}{10}$ **b** $\frac{6}{10} = \frac{3}{5}$ **c** $\frac{8}{10} = \frac{4}{5}$	*1P*
35	**a** $\frac{55}{100} = \frac{11}{20}$ **b** $\frac{72}{100} = \frac{18}{25}$ **c** $\frac{68}{100} = \frac{17}{25}$ **d** $\frac{9}{100}$	*1P*
36	**a** $\frac{6}{100} = \frac{3}{50}$ **b** $\frac{43}{100}$ **c** $\frac{75}{100} = \frac{3}{4}$	*1Q*
37	**a** $\frac{7}{1000}$ **b** $\frac{3}{10\,000}$ **c** $\frac{5}{10\,000} = \frac{1}{2000}$	*1Q*
38	**a** $\frac{1}{200}$ **b** $\frac{11}{200}$ **c** $\frac{35}{200} = \frac{7}{40}$	*1Q*
39	**a** $8\frac{1}{2}$ **b** $22\frac{1}{3}$ **c** $22\frac{3}{5}$	*1R*
40	**a** $\frac{11}{4}$ **b** $\frac{77}{6}$ **c** $\frac{142}{5}$	*1R*
41	**a** $\frac{5}{9}$ **b** $1\frac{1}{14}$ **c** $\frac{2}{5}$	*1S*
42	**a** $1\frac{2}{3}$ **b** $\frac{5}{7}$ **c** $\frac{25}{28}$	*1T*

9. Answers

Chapter 1: A review of basic calculations

Exercise 1A

Multiplication by 10, 100, 1000

1 6.8, 68, 680
2 9.75, 97.5, 975
3 37, 370, 3700
4 56.2, 562, 5620
5 770, 7700, 77 000
6 8250, 82 500, 825 000
7 2, 20, 200
8 0.46, 4.6, 46
9 0.147, 1.47, 14.7
10 0.06, 0.6, 6
11 37.6, 376, 3760
12 6.39, 63.9, 639
13 0.75, 7.5, 75
14 0.8, 8, 80
15 0.03, 0.3, 3
16 0.505, 5.05, 50.5

Exercise 1B

Division by 10, 100, 1000

1 9.84, 0.984, 0.0984
2 0.591, 0.0591, 0.005 91
3 0.26, 0.026, 0.0026
4 30.7, 3.07, 0.307
5 8.2, 0.82, 0.082
6 0.7, 0.07, 0.007
7 0.3, 0.03, 0.003
8 0.75, 0.075, 0.0075
9 6.8, 0.68, 0.068
10 0.229, 0.0229, 0.002 29
11 5.14, 0.514, 0.0514
12 91.6, 9.16, 0.916
13 6.72, 0.672, 0.0672
14 38.7, 3.87, 0.387
15 0.894, 0.0894, 0.008 94
16 0.0707, 0.007 07, 0.000 707

Exercise 1C

Converting metric units

Milligrams:

1 4000
2 8700
3 690
4 20
5 35
6 6
7 655
8 4280

Grams:

9 6
10 7.25
11 0.865
12 0.095
13 0.07
14 0.002
15 0.005
16 0.125

Micrograms:

17 195	**19** 750	**21** 80	**23** 625
18 600	**20** 75	**22** 1	**24** 98

Milligrams:

25 0.825	**27** 0.065	**29** 0.01	**31** 0.2
26 0.75	**28** 0.095	**30** 0.005	**32** 0.03

Millilitres:

33 2000	**35** 1500	**37** 1600	**39** 800
34 30 000	**36** 4500	**38** 2240	**40** 750

Litres:

41 4	**43** 0.625	**45** 0.095	**47** 0.005
42 10	**44** 0.35	**46** 0.06	**48** 0.002

Exercise 1D

1 a 100 mL	**b** 10 mL	**c** 0.1 L
2 a 3 mL	**b** 300 mL	**c** 0.3 L
3 a 50 mL	**b** 5 mL	**c** 0.05 L
4 a 47 mL	**b** 470 mL	**c** 0.47 L
5 a 400 mg	**b** 4 mg	**c** 0.4 g
6 a 60 mg	**b** 600 mg	**c** 0.6 g
7 a 70 mg	**b** 7 mg	**c** 0.07 g
8 a 630 mg	**b** 63 mg	**c** 0.63 g
9 a 2 µg	**b** 20 µg	**c** 0.02 mg
10 a 900 µg	**b** 90 µg	**c** 0.9 mg
11 a 1 µg	**b** 100 µg	**c** 0.1 mg
12 a 580 µg	**b** 58 µg	**c** 0.58 mg
13 a 1500 g	**b** 1050 g	**c** 1.5 kg
14 a 2080 g	**b** 2800 g	**c** 2.8 kg
15 a 950 g	**b** 95 g	**c** 0.95 kg
16 a 3350 g	**b** 3500 g	**c** 3.5 kg

Exercise 1E

Multiplication of decimals

1 45, 4.5, 0.45, 0.45
2 14, 0.14, 0.014, 0.0014
3 12, 0.12, 0.12, 0.0012
4 36, 0.36, 0.0036, 0.0036
5 56, 5.6, 0.56, 0.0056
6 102, 10.2, 1.02, 0.102
7 152, 15.2, 0.152, 0.152
8 46, 0.46, 0.046, 0.0046
9 145, 1.45, 1.45, 1.45
10 93, 0.93, 0.0093, 0.093
11 333, 33.3, 0.333, 0.0333
12 287, 0.287, 0.0287, 2.87
13 192, 0.0192, 0.192, 0.0192
14 616, 6.16, 0.0616, 0.616
15 768, 0.768, 0.0768, 0.0768

Exercise 1F

Diluting solutions
Answers in millimetres (mL):

1	500	11	1035	21	1265
2	450	12	825	22	2700
3	525	13	820	23	2850
4	500	14	775	24	3305
5	625	15	955	25	2850
6	475	16	1650	26	2725
7	800	17	1575	27	2965
8	850	18	1785	28	4350
9	915	19	1350	29	3990
10	950	20	1325	30	3875

Exercise 1G

Factors

1 2, 4, 5
2 3, 4, 12
3 3, 5, 15
4 2, 8, 14
5 3, 4, 12, 15, 20
6 3, 4, 6, 12, 18
7 3, 5, 15, 25
8 5, 17
9 3, 8, 12, 16, 24
10 5, 20, 25

11 4, 9, 12, 18
12 3, 5, 12, 15
13 3, 5, 9, 15
14 4, 8, 12, 16, 18, 24
15 5, 15, 25
16 3, 5, 11, 15
17 5, 7
18 4, 12, 15
19 4, 6, 8, 12, 16
20 6, 14, 15

Exercise 1H

Simplifying fractions I

Part i

1 $\frac{2}{3}$ 6 $\frac{5}{7}$ 11 $\frac{7}{8}$ 16 $\frac{1}{3}$ 21 $\frac{9}{14}$

2 $\frac{5}{7}$ 7 $\frac{5}{6}$ 12 $\frac{2}{3}$ 17 $\frac{2}{3}$ 22 $\frac{4}{5}$

3 $\frac{3}{8}$ 8 $\frac{4}{5}$ 13 $\frac{3}{7}$ 18 $\frac{7}{8}$ 23 $\frac{13}{16}$

4 $\frac{1}{2}$ 9 $\frac{3}{7}$ 14 $\frac{8}{9}$ 19 $\frac{18}{25}$ 24 $\frac{3}{10}$

5 $\frac{3}{4}$ 10 $\frac{3}{10}$ 15 $\frac{2}{5}$ 20 $\frac{5}{11}$ 25 $\frac{4}{9}$

Part ii

1 $\frac{1}{2}$ 5 $\frac{1}{2}$ 9 $\frac{2}{15}$ 13 $\frac{5}{8}$ 17 $\frac{7}{9}$

2 $\frac{3}{8}$ 6 $\frac{5}{12}$ 10 $\frac{8}{35}$ 14 $\frac{3}{4}$ 18 $\frac{3}{4}$

3 $\frac{3}{10}$ 7 $\frac{5}{16}$ 11 $\frac{3}{10}$ 15 $\frac{11}{16}$ 19 $\frac{17}{24}$

4 $\frac{1}{4}$ 8 $\frac{1}{4}$ 12 $\frac{4}{25}$ 16 $\frac{4}{9}$ 20 $\frac{13}{30}$

Exercise 1I

Simplifying fractions II

1 $\frac{3}{5}$	**7** $\frac{13}{15}$	**13** $\frac{2}{3}$	**19** $\frac{2}{3}$	**25** $\frac{2}{3}$	**31** $\frac{5}{6}$
2 $\frac{2}{3}$	**8** $\frac{2}{3}$	**14** $\frac{2}{5}$	**20** $\frac{3}{4}$	**26** $\frac{8}{15}$	**32** $\frac{1}{6}$
3 $\frac{3}{4}$	**9** $\frac{2}{5}$	**15** $\frac{9}{10}$	**21** $\frac{9}{10}$	**27** $\frac{5}{6}$	**33** $\frac{3}{20}$
4 $\frac{5}{12}$	**10** $\frac{3}{4}$	**16** $\frac{3}{5}$	**22** $\frac{3}{4}$	**28** $\frac{14}{25}$	**34** $\frac{3}{8}$
5 $\frac{2}{3}$	**11** $\frac{5}{8}$	**17** $\frac{9}{10}$	**23** $\frac{15}{16}$	**29** $\frac{4}{5}$	**35** $\frac{3}{10}$
6 $\frac{5}{6}$	**12** $\frac{3}{8}$	**18** $\frac{6}{25}$	**24** $\frac{2}{5}$	**30** $\frac{7}{10}$	**36** $\frac{11}{16}$

Exercise 1J

Rounding-off decimal numbers

Part i

1 0.9	**5** 0.6	**9** 2.4	**13** 1.1
2 0.5	**6** 1.0	**10** 1.1	**14** 3.0
3 0.9	**7** 1.6	**11** 0.2	**15** 1.0
4 0.7	**8** 1.2	**12** 2.7	**16** 0.8

Part ii

1 0.33	**5** 0.14	**9** 2.71	**13** 0.63
2 1.67	**6** 0.13	**10** 1.29	**14** 0.78
3 0.88	**7** 0.92	**11** 0.64	**15** 2.43
4 0.83	**8** 1.57	**12** 0.22	**16** 1.86

Part iii

1 0.486	**5** 1.529	**9** 0.816	**13** 3.091
2 0.955	**6** 0.311	**10** 1.120	**14** 0.165
3 0.606	**7** 2.859	**11** 0.165	**15** 2.780
4 1.415	**8** 0.170	**12** 2.963	**16** 1.758

Exercise 1K

Vulgar fraction to a decimal I

1 0.5	**7** 0.125	**13** 0.04	**19** 0.275
2 0.25	**8** 0.875	**14** 0.32	**20** 0.675
3 0.75	**9** 0.05	**15** 0.68	**21** 0.02
4 0.2	**10** 0.35	**16** 0.88	**22** 0.86
5 0.6	**11** 0.65	**17** 0.025	**23** 0.0125
6 0.8	**12** 0.95	**18** 0.225	**24** 0.7625

Exercise 1L

Vulgar fraction to a decimal II

Part i

1 0.3	**3** 0.3	**5** 0.2	**7** 0.5
2 0.8	**4** 0.7	**6** 0.3	**8** 0.9

Part ii

1 0.67	**3** 0.86	**5** 0.89	**7** 0.91
2 0.17	**4** 0.44	**6** 0.36	**8** 0.42

Part iii

1 0.033	**3** 0.117	**5** 0.129	**7** 0.011
2 0.567	**4** 0.517	**6** 0.757	**8** 0.256

Exercise 1M

Vulgar fraction to a percentage

1 50%	**11** 90%	**21** 28%	**31** $87\frac{1}{2}$%
2 25%	**12** 5%	**22** 44%	**32** $16\frac{2}{3}$%
3 75%	**13** 15%	**23** 52%	**33** $83\frac{1}{3}$%
4 20%	**14** 45%	**24** 68%	**34** $11\frac{1}{9}$%
5 40%	**15** 55%	**25** 76%	**35** $44\frac{4}{9}$%
6 60%	**16** 65%	**26** 92%	**36** $77\frac{7}{9}$%
7 80%	**17** 85%	**27** $33\frac{1}{3}$%	**37** $2\frac{1}{2}$%
8 10%	**18** 95%	**28** $66\frac{2}{3}$%	**38** $7\frac{1}{2}$%
9 30%	**19** 4%	**29** $12\frac{1}{2}$%	**39** $22\frac{1}{2}$%
10 70%	**20** 12%	**30** $62\frac{1}{2}$%	**40** $27\frac{1}{2}$%

Exercise 1N

Dilution ratios

Part i

1 1 in 3	**4** 1 in 11	**7** 1 in 31	**10** 1 in 201
2 1 in 6	**5** 1 in 16	**8** 1 in 51	**11** 1 in 251
3 1 in 8	**6** 1 in 26	**9** 1 in 101	**12** 1 in 501

Part ii

1 1 : 1	**4** 1 : 6	**7** 1 : 19	**10** 1 : 49
2 1 : 2	**5** 1 : 9	**8** 1 : 24	**11** 1 : 99
3 1 : 4	**6** 1 : 14	**9** 1 : 39	**12** 1 : 199

Part iii (millilitres)

1 25, 20	**5** 70, 60	**9** 150, 129
2 75, 50	**6** 55, 50	**10** 143, 125
3 60, 50	**7** 133, 100	**11** 250, 222
4 200, 150	**8** 188, 150	**12** 556, 500

Exercise 1O

Ratio to percentage

1 50%	**17** 33.33%	**33** 0.13%
2 25%	**18** 16.67%	**34** 0.11%
3 20%	**19** 14.29%	**35** Relationships:
4 10%	**20** 12.5%	1 in 20 = $\frac{1}{10}$ of 1 in 2
5 5%	**21** 11.11%	1 in 200 = $\frac{1}{10}$ of 1 in 20
6 4%	**22** 8.33%	1 in 30 = $\frac{1}{10}$ of 1 in 3
7 2%	**23** 6.67%	1 in 300 = $\frac{1}{10}$ of 1 in 30
8 1%	**24** 3.33%	**36** 33.33%
9 0.5%	**25** 1.67%	**37** 25%
10 0.4%	**26** 1.43%	**38** 16.67%
11 0.25%	**27** 1.33%	**39** 14.29%
12 0.1%	**28** 1.25%	**40** 12.5%
13 0.05%	**29** 1.11%	**41** 11.11%
14 0.04%	**30** 0.33%	**42** 10%
15 0.02%	**31** 0.25%	
16 0.01%	**32** 0.14%	

Exercise 1P

Decimal fraction to vulgar fraction

Part i

1 $\frac{1}{10}$	**3** $\frac{3}{10}$	**5** $\frac{3}{5}$	**7** $\frac{4}{5}$
2 $\frac{1}{5}$	**4** $\frac{1}{2}$	**6** $\frac{7}{10}$	**8** $\frac{9}{10}$

Part ii

1 $\frac{6}{25}$	**9** $\frac{19}{20}$	**17** $\frac{4}{25}$	**25** $\frac{9}{50}$	**33** $\frac{41}{100}$
2 $\frac{23}{50}$	**10** $\frac{11}{20}$	**18** $\frac{83}{100}$	**26** $\frac{69}{100}$	**34** $\frac{2}{25}$
3 $\frac{77}{100}$	**11** $\frac{3}{100}$	**19** $\frac{9}{20}$	**27** $\frac{12}{25}$	**35** $\frac{16}{25}$
4 $\frac{13}{100}$	**12** $\frac{18}{25}$	**20** $\frac{24}{25}$	**28** $\frac{1}{20}$	**36** $\frac{7}{25}$
5 $\frac{7}{20}$	**13** $\frac{13}{20}$	**21** $\frac{3}{4}$	**29** $\frac{17}{20}$	**37** $\frac{79}{100}$
6 $\frac{81}{100}$	**14** $\frac{1}{4}$	**22** $\frac{13}{50}$	**30** $\frac{23}{25}$	**38** $\frac{19}{50}$
7 $\frac{33}{50}$	**15** $\frac{9}{25}$	**23** $\frac{39}{100}$	**31** $\frac{57}{100}$	**39** $\frac{99}{100}$
8 $\frac{1}{100}$	**16** $\frac{29}{50}$	**24** $\frac{53}{100}$	**32** $\frac{87}{100}$	**40** $\frac{3}{20}$

Exercise 1Q

Percentage to vulgar fraction

Part i

1 $\frac{1}{50}$	**4** $\frac{1}{20}$	**7** $\frac{3}{25}$	**10** $\frac{3}{10}$	**13** $\frac{9}{20}$
2 $\frac{3}{100}$	**5** $\frac{7}{100}$	**8** $\frac{3}{20}$	**11** $\frac{7}{20}$	**14** $\frac{1}{2}$
3 $\frac{1}{25}$	**6** $\frac{1}{10}$	**9** $\frac{1}{5}$	**12** $\frac{2}{5}$	**15** $\frac{9}{10}$

Part ii

1 $\frac{1}{1000}$	**4** $\frac{1}{200}$	**7** $\frac{1}{125}$	**10** $\frac{1}{5000}$	**13** $\frac{3}{5000}$
2 $\frac{1}{500}$	**5** $\frac{3}{500}$	**8** $\frac{9}{1000}$	**11** $\frac{1}{2500}$	**14** $\frac{7}{10\,000}$
3 $\frac{1}{250}$	**6** $\frac{7}{1000}$	**9** $\frac{1}{10\,000}$	**12** $\frac{1}{2000}$	**15** $\frac{9}{10\,000}$

Part iii

1 $\frac{1}{200}$	**3** $\frac{1}{40}$	**5** $\frac{3}{40}$
2 $\frac{3}{200}$	**4** $\frac{9}{200}$	**6** $\frac{1}{8}$

Exercise 1R

Mixed numbers and improper fractions

Part i

1 $2\frac{1}{2}$	**5** $4\frac{5}{6}$	**9** $25\frac{1}{2}$	**13** $15\frac{5}{6}$	**17** $26\frac{3}{5}$
2 $3\frac{2}{3}$	**6** $5\frac{1}{7}$	**10** $21\frac{2}{3}$	**14** $14\frac{3}{7}$	**18** $23\frac{5}{6}$
3 $4\frac{1}{4}$	**7** $4\frac{5}{8}$	**11** $17\frac{3}{4}$	**15** $14\frac{1}{8}$	**19** $22\frac{3}{7}$
4 $4\frac{2}{5}$	**8** $5\frac{4}{9}$	**12** $17\frac{1}{5}$	**16** $13\frac{8}{9}$	**20** $18\frac{4}{9}$

Part ii

1 $\frac{3}{2}$	**5** $\frac{7}{2}$	**9** $\frac{67}{6}$	**13** $\frac{45}{2}$	**17** $\frac{185}{6}$
2 $\frac{4}{3}$	**6** $\frac{14}{3}$	**10** $\frac{93}{7}$	**14** $\frac{74}{3}$	**18** $\frac{228}{7}$
3 $\frac{7}{4}$	**7** $\frac{25}{4}$	**11** $\frac{133}{8}$	**15** $\frac{111}{4}$	**19** $\frac{283}{8}$
4 $\frac{13}{5}$	**8** $\frac{49}{5}$	**12** $\frac{155}{9}$	**16** $\frac{146}{5}$	**20** $\frac{347}{9}$

Exercise 1S

Multiplication of vulgar fractions

1 $\frac{1}{5}$	**10** $\frac{3}{20}$	**19** $\frac{9}{10}$	**28** $\frac{3}{16}$
2 $\frac{5}{24}$	**11** $\frac{4}{9}$	**20** $\frac{9}{32}$	**29** $\frac{2}{15}$
3 $\frac{5}{9}$	**12** $\frac{1}{18}$	**21** 1	**30** $\frac{1}{5}$
4 $\frac{1}{6}$	**13** $\frac{11}{42}$	**22** $\frac{1}{135}$	**31** $\frac{27}{32}$
5 $1\frac{2}{3}$	**14** $\frac{3}{140}$	**23** $\frac{7}{18}$	**32** $\frac{1}{18}$
6 $\frac{3}{50}$	**15** $\frac{20}{21}$	**24** $\frac{5}{27}$	**33** $\frac{1}{360}$
7 $\frac{3}{5}$	**16** $\frac{12}{35}$	**25** $\frac{7}{15}$	**34** $\frac{7}{72}$
8 $\frac{9}{20}$	**17** $\frac{5}{28}$	**26** $\frac{7}{16}$	**35** $\frac{21}{160}$
9 $\frac{5}{6}$	**18** $\frac{1}{16}$	**27** $\frac{4}{27}$	**36** $\frac{121}{160}$

Exercise 1T

Division by a vulgar fraction

1 $\frac{2}{3}$	**10** $3\frac{3}{4}$	**19** $\frac{10}{21}$	**28** $\frac{1}{3}$
2 $1\frac{1}{2}$	**11** $\frac{3}{5}$	**20** $1\frac{5}{7}$	**29** $2\frac{2}{3}$
3 $1\frac{1}{3}$	**12** $\frac{2}{3}$	**21** $\frac{3}{14}$	**30** $\frac{8}{9}$
4 $\frac{3}{5}$	**13** $\frac{2}{3}$	**22** $1\frac{1}{7}$	**31** $1\frac{1}{9}$
5 4	**14** $1\frac{1}{5}$	**23** $\frac{1}{7}$	**32** $1\frac{1}{3}$
6 $1\frac{1}{2}$	**15** $\frac{3}{14}$	**24** $\frac{5}{12}$	**33** $\frac{7}{10}$
7 $\frac{1}{2}$	**16** $2\frac{1}{12}$	**25** $\frac{3}{4}$	**34** $\frac{9}{25}$
8 $\frac{5}{16}$	**17** $1\frac{1}{7}$	**26** $1\frac{3}{4}$	**35** $\frac{4}{5}$
9 $\frac{9}{10}$	**18** $\frac{5}{14}$	**27** $\frac{5}{9}$	**36** $1\frac{1}{2}$

Chapter 2: Drug dosages for injection

All answers are in millilitres (mL)

Exercise 2A

1 less than 1 mL
2 more than 2 mL
3 less than 5 mL
4 less than 2 mL
5 equal to 3 mL
6 less than 2 mL
7 more than 1 mL

Exercise 2B

1 0.8	**3** 0.9	**5** 1.3	**7** 1.5
2 1.4	**4** 4	**6** 1.7	**8** 1.6

Exercise 2C

1 1.5	**4** 4	**6** 0.2	**8** 1.6
2 3.2	**5** 0.8	**7** 1.3	**9** 0.55
3 0.5			

Exercise 2D

1 1.6	**4** 0.25	**6** 1.5	**8** 0.6
2 1.2	**5** 2.4	**7** 0.6	**9** 0.8
3 0.75			

Exercise 2E

1 6.7	**4** 0.67	**6** 0.43	**8** 1.8
2 1.3	**5** 0.67	**7** 1.4	**9** 1.3
3 0.83			

Exercise 2F

1 0.8	**6** 1.6	**11** 4	**16** 6.3
2 0.28	**7** 1.2	**12** 0.3	**17** 1.7
3 7	**8** 0.8	**13** 1.5	**18** 0.75
4 0.6	**9** 3	**14** 7.5	**19** 1.5
5 0.35	**10** 3.6	**15** 0.75	**20** 0.72

Exercise 2G   [Need to *include* mL or units]

1 i $\frac{1}{100}$ mL or 0.01 mL
   ii 0.38 mL
   iii 0.73 mL

2 i $\frac{1}{10}$ mL or 0.1 mL
   ii 1.2 mL
   iii 2.15 mL

3 i 2 units
   ii 40 units
   iii 75 units

4 i 0.2 mL
   ii 2.2 mL
   iii 4.5 mL

Answers to chapter revisions

If you make an error in answering any of the questions in the chapter revision exercises, then refer back to the worked examples in the corresponding exercises and also to the relevant arithmetic skills as listed in brackets after each answer.

Chapter 2   **Revision**

All answers in mL. Volumes more than 1 mL are rounded off to one decimal place, volumes less than 1 mL to two decimal places.

 1 less than 1 mL [2A]
 2 1.4 [2B, 2C, 2D: 1H, 1I, 1K, 1R, 1S]
 3 2.4 [2B, 2C, 2D: 1H, 1I, 1K, 1S]
 4 0.4 [2B, 2C, 2D: 1H, 1I, 1K, 1R, 1S]
 5 1.1 [2B, 2C, 2D: 1H, 1I, 1K, 1R, 1S]
 6 2.8 [2B, 2C, 2D: 1H, 1I, 1K, 1R, 1S]
 7 0.45 [2B, 2C, 2D: 1H, 1I, 1K, 1S]
 8 0.9 [2B, 2C, 2D: 1A, 1C, 1D, 1H, 1I, 1K, 1S]
 9 6.3 [2E: 1H, 1I, 1J, 1K, 1R, 1S]
10 0.67 [2E: 1H, 1J, 1K, 1S]

Chapter 3:   Dosages of tablets and mixtures

Exercise 3A   *Number of tablets*

1 3   **3** $1\frac{1}{2}$ **5** 3   **7** $1\frac{1}{2}$
2 2   **4** $\frac{1}{2}$ **6** $\frac{1}{2}$ **8** $\frac{1}{2}$

Exercise 3B

1 a 2 mg + 2 mg (2 tabs)
  b 5 mg + 2 mg + 2 mg (3 tabs)
  c 10 mg + 2 mg (2 tabs)
  d 10 mg + 5 mg (2 tabs)
2 a 5 mg + 2 mg (2 tabs)
  b 5 mg + 2 mg + 2 mg (3 tabs)
  c 10 mg + 5 mg (2 tabs)
  d 10 mg + 10 mg (2 tabs)
3 a 120 mg + 80 mg (2 tabs); or 160 mg + 40 mg (2 tabs)
  b 120 mg + 120 mg; or 160 mg + 80 mg (2 tabs)
  c 160 mg + 120 mg (2 tabs)
  d 160 mg + 160 mg (2 tabs)

4 **a** 5 mg + 1 mg (2 tabs)
   b 5 mg + 2 mg + 1 mg (3 tabs)
   c 5 mg + 2 mg + 2 mg (3 tabs)
   d 5 mg + 5 mg + 1 mg (3 tabs)
5 **a** 6 mg + 3 mg (2 tabs)
   b 12 mg + 3 mg (2 tabs)
   c 12 mg + 6 mg (2 tabs)
   d 12 mg + 6 mg + 3 mg (3 tabs)
6 **a** 25 mg + 10 mg (2 tabs)
   b 50 mg + 10 mg (2 tabs)
   c 50 mg + 25 mg (2 tabs)
   d 100 mg + 10 mg + 10 mg (3 tabs)

Exercise 3C *Volume in mL*

| **1** 20 | **3** 30 | **5** 25 | **7** 20 | **9** 24 |
| **2** 20 | **4** 20 | **6** 30 | **8** 7 | **10** 32 |

Chapter 3 Revision

1 2 [3A: 1H, 1I, 1S]

2 $\frac{1}{2}$ [3A: 1A, 1E, 1H, 1S]

3 $1\frac{1}{2}$ [3A: 1H, 1R, 1S]

4 **a** 2 mg + 1 mg (2 tabs)
   b 5 mg + 2 mg (2 tabs)
   c 10 mg + 2 mg + 1 mg (3 tabs)
   d 10 mg + 5 mg + 1 mg (3 tabs) [3B]

5 Shaken thoroughly

6 15 mL [3C: 1H, 1I, 1S]

7 25 mL [3C: 1H, 1I, 1S]

8 16 mL [3C: 1H, 1I, 1S]

9 15 mL [3C: 1H, 1S]

Chapter 4: Dilution and strengths of solutions

Exercise 4A

1   **a**   1 in 1000   **b**   1 in 100   **c**   1 in 10

2   **a**   1 in 2   **b**   1 in 4   **c**   1 in 5
    d   1 in 10   **e**   1 in 20   **f**   1 in 40
    g   1 in 50   **h**   1 in 200   **i**   1 in 500
    j   1 in 1000

3   **a**   1 in 25   **b**   4%

4   **a**   1 in 20   **b**   5%

5   $1\frac{1}{4}\% = 1.25\%$

6   **a**   0.05%   **b**   0.02%

Exercise 4B   *All answers in mL*

1   100; 100   5   50; 450

2   17.5; 17.5   6   250; 750

3   5; 195   7   **a**   50; 950   **b**   100; 1900   **c**   60; 1140

4   12.5; 487.5   8   **a**   100; 400   **b**   150; 600   **c**   500; 2000

Exercise 4C   *All answers in mL*

1   200; 800   5   120; 480   8   40; 1960

2   250; 1250   6   600; 2400   9   7; 693

3   250; 250   7   125; 2375   10   400; 400

4   750; 750

Exercise 4D   *All answers in mL*

1   40; 760   5   50; 950   8   125; 875

2   150; 1350   6   30; 1170   9   37.5; 262.5

3   50; 4950   7   3.5; 346.5   10   6.25; 93.75

4   250; 2250

Exercise 4E

1   100 mg

2   50 mg

3   **a**   30 g   **b**   75 g   **c**   10 g

4 **a** 100 g   **b** 75 g   **c** 84 g
5 15 g
6 **a** 100 mL   **b** 125 mL
7 **a** 5%   **b** 1.5%   **c** 0.2%
8 17.5 g
9 0.15 g or 150 mg

Chapter 4   Revision

1 **a** 1 in 20 or $\frac{1}{20}$ **b** 5% [4A: 1H, 1I, 1M, 1N, 1S]
2 40 g [4E: 1H, 1I, 1Q, 1S]
3 15 mg [4E: 1C, 1H, 1I, 1Q, 1S]
4 150 mL; 2850 mL [4B: 1A, 1C, 1H, 1I, 1S]
5 300 mL; 900 mL [4B: 1H, 1I, 1S]
6 40 mL; 560 mL [4C: 1C, 1F, 1H, 1I, 1N, 1S, 1T]
7 9 mL; 891 mL [4C: 1C, 1F, 1H, 1I, 1N, 1Q, 1S, 1T]
8 35 mL; 1365 mL [4D: 1C, 1H, 1I, 1Q, 1S, 1T]
9 75 mL; 525 mL [4D: 1H, 1I, 1S]

Chapter 5:   Intravenous infusion

Exercise 5A

1 **a** 80 mL   **b** 320 mL
  c 480 mL

2 **a** 105 mL   **b** 175 mL
  c 420 mL

3 **a** 90 mL   **b** 150 mL
  c 720 mL

4 20 hours

5 $12\frac{1}{2}$ hours or 12 h 30 min

6 $6\frac{2}{3}$ hours or 6 h 40 min

7 $\frac{2}{3}$ h = 40 min

Exercise 5B

1 125 mL/h

2 125 mL/h

3 $71\frac{3}{7} \Rightarrow 72$ mL/h

4 $133\frac{1}{3} \Rightarrow 134$ mL/h

5 $187\frac{1}{2} \Rightarrow 188$ mL/h

Exercise 5C

1 5 hours

2 10 hours

3 $8\frac{1}{3}$ hours or 8 h 20 min

4 $6\frac{2}{3}$ hours or 6 h 40 min

5 $6\frac{1}{4}$ hours or 6 h 15 min

Exercise 5D

1 25 drops/min

2 $20\frac{5}{6} \Rightarrow 21$ drops/min

3 $10\frac{5}{12} \Rightarrow 11$ drops/min

4 $13\frac{8}{9} \Rightarrow 14$ drops/min

5 25 drops/min

6 50 drops/min

7 90 drops/min

Exercise 5E

1 25 drops/min

2 $31\frac{1}{4} \Rightarrow 32$ drops/min

3 $37\frac{1}{2} \Rightarrow 38$ drops/min

4 $12\frac{1}{2} \Rightarrow 13$ drops/min

5 $27\frac{7}{9} \Rightarrow 28$ drops/min

6 $20\frac{5}{6} \Rightarrow 21$ drops/min

Exercise 5F

1 1800 mL

2 6 h + 7 h = 13 hours

3 Total running time = 5 h + $2\frac{1}{2}$ h = $7\frac{1}{2}$ hours or 7 h 30 min

∴ Finishing time = 0800 h + 7 h 30 min = 1530 hours

4 Total running time = 10 h + 8 h = 18 hours
∴ Finishing time = 0430 h + 18 h = 2230 hours
5 110 mL/h
6 55 mL/h

Exercise 5G   *All answers in kilojoules*

1	800	**5**	0 (no carbohydrate)
2	2000	**6**	480
3	1600	**7**	0 (no carbohydrate)
4	1600	**8**	400

Chapter 5   Revision

1 **a** 110 mL   **b** 275 mL   **c** 605 mL [5A]

2 $8\frac{1}{3}$ hours or 8 h 20 min [5A: 1C, 1H, 1I, 1R]

3 75 mL/h [5B: 1C, 1H, 1I]

4 $90\frac{10}{11} \Rightarrow$ 91 mL/h [5B: 1C, 1D, 1R]

5 $6\frac{1}{4}$ hours or 6 h 15 min [5C: 1H, 1I, 1R, 1S]

6 50 drops/min [5D, 5E: 1C, 1D, 1H, 1I, 1S]

7 $20\frac{5}{6} \Rightarrow$ 21 drops/min [5D, 5E: 1C, 1H, 1I, 1R, 1S]

8 1620 mL [5F]

9 6 h + 11 h = 17 h [5F: 1C, 1H, 1I]

10 Total running time = 8 h + 11 h = 19 hours
∴ Finishing time = 0300 h + 19 h = 2200 hours
[5F: 1C, 1H, 1I]

11 115 mL/h [5F: 1C, 1H, 1I]

12 1200 kJ [5G: 1B, 1C]

Chapter 6:   Paediatric dosages (body weight)

Exercise 6A   *All answers in milligrams*

1	120	**4**	250	**7**	900
2	150	**5**	200	**8**	240
3	90	**6**	225	**9**	540

Exercise 6B   *All answers in millilitres*

1	0.4	**6**	0.72	**11**	1.2	**16**	1.5
2	0.4	**7**	0.4	**12**	0.3	**17**	1.0
3	0.8	**8**	0.75	**13**	0.25	**18**	0.8
4	0.75	**9**	0.48	**14**	0.6	**19**	0.6
5	0.5	**10**	1.2	**15**	0.65	**20**	0.8

Exercise 6C   *All answers in millilitres*

1	3.5	**4**	9	**7**	14	**10**	$6\frac{2}{3}$ or 6.7
2	12.5	**5**	2.5	**8**	3	**11**	0.5
3	6	**6**	8	**9**	4	**12**	4

Chapter 6   **Revision**

1 275 mg [6A]

2 285 mg [6A]

3 180 mg [6A]

4 $\frac{3}{5}$ mL or 0.6 mL
    [6B: 1H, 1I, 1K, 1S]

5 0.96 mL
    [6B: 1C, 1H, 1I, 1K, 1S]

6 1.8 mL
    [6B: 1H, 1I, 1K, 1R, 1S]

7 7.5 mL
    [6C: 1H, 1I, 1K, 1R, 1S]

8 8 mL [6C: 1H, 1I, 1S]

9 12 mL [6C: 1H, 1I, 1S]

Chapter 7:   Paediatric dosages (surface area)

Exercise 7A   *All answers in m²*

1	**a**	0.35	**4**	**a**	0.57	**7**	**a**	0.51
	b	0.40		**b**	0.64		**b**	0.53
2	**a**	0.43	**5**	**a**	0.31	**8**	**a**	0.59
	b	0.48		**b**	0.32		**b**	0.61
3	**a**	0.51	**6**	**a**	0.43			
	b	0.57		**b**	0.45			

Exercise 7B   *All answers in mL*

1	1.2	**2**	1.8	**3**	2.7	**4**	3.9	**5**	0.96

Chapter 7 Revision

1 0.68 m² [7A only]
2 0.75 m² [7A]
3 0.82 m² [7A]
4 0,90 m² [7A]

5 1.6 mL
[7B: 1A, 1H, 1I, 1K, 1R, 1S]
6 10.5 mL
[7B: 1E, 1H, 1I, 1K, 1R, 1S]

Chapter 8: Summary exercises

Summary exercise I

1 more than 5 mL
2 4.5 mL
3 0.5 mL
4 $1\frac{1}{2}$ tablets
5 **a** 2 mg + 2 mg [2 tabs]
  b 5 mg + 2 mg + 1 mg
  [3 tabs] **c** 10 mg + 2 mg
  [2 tabs]
6 14.4 mL
7 $\frac{1}{8}$ or 1 in 8
8 **a** 250 mL **b** 4750 mL
9 **a** 500 mL **b** 2000 mL
10 **a** 150 mL **b** 1050 mL
11 50 g

12 **a** 75 mL **b** 125 mL
  c 300 mL
13 $83\frac{1}{3} \Rightarrow 84$ mL/h
14 $21\frac{7}{8} \Rightarrow 22$ drops/min
15 5 h + $7\frac{1}{2}$ h = $12\frac{1}{2}$ hours
  or 12 h 30 min
16 800 kJ
17 225 mg/dose
18 0.7 mL
19 0.35 mL
20 2.5 mL
21 0.43 m²
22 0.99 mL

Summary exercise II

1 less than 3 mL
2 0.9 mL
3 $\frac{1}{2}$ tablet
4 **a** 50 mg + 10 mg [2 tabs]
  b 50 mg + 25 mg + 10 mg
  [3tabs] **c** 100 mg + 10 mg
  [2 tabs]
5 18 mL
6 0.5%
7 4%
8 **a** 15 mL   **b** 585 mL
9 **a** 20 mL   **b** 780 mL
10 120 mL Savlon; 2280 mL
   water

11 75 g
12 $12\frac{1}{2}$ hours or 12 h 30 min
13 $55\frac{5}{9} \Rightarrow 56$ mL/h
14 $6\frac{1}{4}$ hours or 6 h 15 min
15 12 h + 5 h = 17 hours
16 1280 kJ
17 160 mg/dose
18 1.4 mL
19 6 mL
20 7 mL
21 0.58 m^2
22 0.9 mL